Clinical Orthopaedic Examination

Clinical Orthopaedic Examination

Ronald McRae FRCS

Consultant Orthopaedic Surgeon, Southern General Hospital,
Glasgow. Honorary Clinical Lecturer in Orthopaedics, University of
Glasgow. Director of Studies and Lecturer in Anatomy, Glasgow
School of Chiropody. Fellow of the British Orthopaedic Association
and Member of the Institute of Medical and Biological Illustration

With original drawings by the author

SECOND EDITION

CHURCHILL LIVINGSTONE
EDINBURGH LONDON MELBOURNE AND NEW YORK 1983

CHURCHILL LIVINGSTONE
Medical Division of Longman Group Limited

Distributed in the United States of America by
Churchill Livingstone Inc., 1560 Broadway,
New York, N.Y. 10036, and by associated
companies, branches and representatives
throughout the world.

First edition 1976
Second edition 1983

ISBN 0 443 02447 2

British Library Cataloguing in Publication Data
McRae, Ronald
 Clinical orthopaedic examination.—2nd ed.
 1. Orthopedia—Diagnosis
 2. Physical diagnosis
 I. Title
 617'.3   RD734

Library of Congress Cataloguing in Publication Data
McRae, Ronald.
 Clinical orthopaedic examination.
 Includes bibliographical references and index.
 ı1. Orthopedia—Diagnosis. 2. Musculo-skeletal system—
Examination. I. Title.
[DNLM: 1. Bone diseases—Diagnosis—Atlases.
2. Joint diseases—Diagnosis—Atlases.
3. Orthopedics—Atlases. WE 17 M174c]
RD734.M3 1983   617'.3   82-4391
                               AACR2

Printed in Hong Kong
by Hing Yip Printing Co

Preface

The ability to make a good clinical examination can only be mastered by practice, and I have no doubt that the basic techniques are best learned by performance under supervision. Unfortunately the size of student classes in relation to teaching staff and the not infrequent dearth of an adequate range of suitable clinical cases makes this ideal difficult to achieve in practice. Many students may acquire only a sketchy knowledge of the techniques of examination which are fundamental to diagnosis and treatment. It is hoped that this book may help to fill some of these inevitable gaps until sound practice based on experience is achieved.

The text

It is assumed that the value of good history-taking is appreciated and practised.

Patients parade their complaints on an anatomical basis, and the text has been arranged accordingly. The emphasis in each section is on the common rather than the rare conditions to be found in the region. Although this approach is open to criticism, it is nevertheless true to say that while the obscure will tax the most experienced, the most frequent mistake is a failure to diagnose the common. An encyclopaedic text, commendable on the ground of completeness, may nevertheless often confuse, especially where no indication is given of incidence of the conditions observed. I have purposely avoided detail, and where this is required a fuller orthopaedic textbook must be consulted. In some areas too I have made deliberate simplification where a blight of terminology suggests the independence of a number of conditions which cannot be distinguished by symptomatology or investigation.

The illustrations

The illustrations dealing with the practical aspects of clinical examination have been arranged in an essentially linear sequence following the traditional lines of inspection, palpation, and the examination of movements and pertinent anatomical structures. In practice, this logical order is often altered by the experienced examiner to avoid undue movement of the patient. It must be stressed that not all the tests described need be carried out routinely. Many are performed only when a specific condition is suspected, and it is assumed that this will be obvious to the reader. In particular, in any joint assessment, it is necessary to discover if there is any restriction of movement; in many cases simple screening tests will suffice, and these are included in most sections. The more detailed examination and recording of movement are generally reserved for cases under lengthy continuous observation and for medico-legal work.

Radiographic examination plays an essential part in the investigation of most orthopaedic cases, and to aid the inexperienced I have made some observations regarding the views normally taken and how they may be interpreted. Only a fraction of the possible pathology can be illustrated in a small work, but again I have concentrated on the common; and while line drawings are not a substitute for full size radiographs, I hope their simplicity will nevertheless be helpful.

The spatial requirements of the captions have set some restriction on their content; this discipline has resulted in brevity at the expense in places of completeness. Nevertheless, wherever possible I have tried to show not only how each test should be carried out, but also its significance.

In the second edition the opportunity has been taken of including normal radiographs in each section, and a number of additional examples of geometric analysis of radiographs have been described. Certain captions have been expanded, and the guides to the normal ranges of joint movement have been adjusted in agreement with recently published work. The text has been rewritten in many places to conform with current opinion. Some new tests have been illustrated and an index added.

Conventions and references

Where two limbs are illustrated, the pathology is shown on the patient's *right* side.

Where several conditions are described, and one representative illustration only is given, it refers to the *first* condition mentioned.

Cross references refer to the illustration number in the appropriate section.

When joint movements are being considered, the patient's normal side should if possible be used for comparison. Angular measurement is an approximation, and the figures quoted are in most cases values rounded to the nearest five degrees from figures published by the American Academy of Orthopaedic Surgeons[1], Kapandji[2], Lusted & Keats[3] or Boone & Azen[4].

Glasgow, 1983   R. McR.

1   American Academy of Orthopaedic Surgeons 1965 Joint motion: method of measuring and recording. Churchill Livingstone, Edinburgh
2   Kapandji A 1982 The physiology of the joints, 5th edn. Churchill Livingstone, Edinburgh
3   Lusted L B, Keats T E 1972 Atlas of roentgenographic measurement. Year Book Medical Publishers, London
4   Boone C D, Azen P S 1979 Journal of Bone and Joint Surgery 61A/5:756–9

Contents

1 Segmental and Peripheral Nerves of the Upper Limb

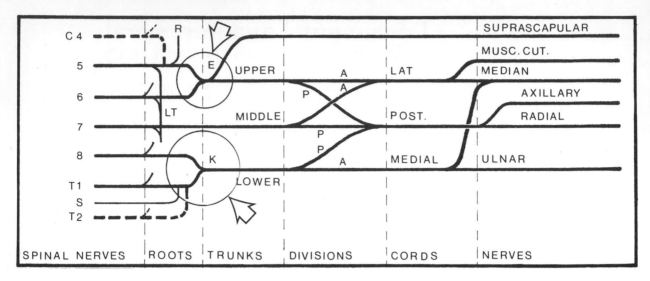

1. *Brachial Plexus:* The *roots* of the brachial plexus are formed by the *anterior* rami of C5–T1 with occasional contributions from C4 and T2. Sympathetic fibres are carried in by T1. The three posterior divisions form the posterior cord. Two anterior divisions form the lateral cord, and the remaining anterior division forms the medial cord. *Note:* (1) In Erb's (*upper obstetrical*) *Palsy* (E) the C5–6 roots are affected, but the nerve to rhomboids (R) and the long thoracic nerve are spared. (2) In Klumpke's (lower obstetrical) Palsy (K) the C8–T1 roots are involved, usually with the sympathetic inflow. 80% of birth injuries to the plexus make a full recovery by 13 months, and persisting severe sensory or motor deficits in the hand are rare. A number are initially accompanied by *facial nerve palsy.* (3) *In traumatic plexus lesions in adults,* the following patterns of root involvement are common: (a) C5–6 (Erb type) (b) C5, 6, 7 (c) C5–T1 (this pattern has the poorest prognosis). If the lesion is in continuity, spontaneous recovery may occur. Repair is sometimes feasible where tearing of roots has occurred distal to the dural pouches, and myelography may be helpful in establishing this. Sparing of serratus anterior and the rhomboids indicates a distal injury; Horner's syndrome, avulsion of a cervical transverse process (X-ray cervical spine), paralysis of half the diaphragm (X-ray chest) suggest root avulsion and are poor prognostic signs.

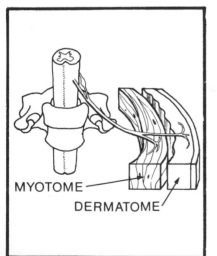

2. *Segmental distribution:* Where you suspect nerve root rather than main nerve involvement (e.g. in cervical spondylosis, spinal and plexus injuries) you must examine myotomes and dermatomes. These are the muscle masses and areas of skin supplied by single spinal nerves.

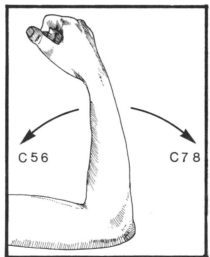

3. *Myotomes* (1) Normally 2 roots produce movement of a joint in one direction and 2 in the other. This is true at the elbow (but modified elsewhere) (e.g. weakness of biceps, absent biceps jerk, indicates C5, 6 involvement; weakness of triceps, absent triceps jerk, C7, 8).

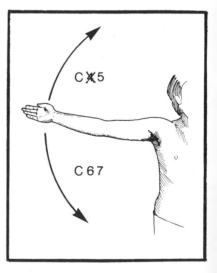

4. *Myotomes* (2) C4 control of the shoulder has been suppressed. Abduction is controlled by C5 alone (deltoid, supraspinatus, etc.). Adduction is controlled by C6, 7 (pectoralis major, etc.).

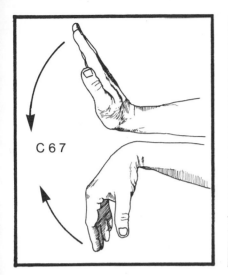

5. *Myotomes* (3) At the wrist, both dorsiflexion and palmar flexion are controlled by C6, 7.

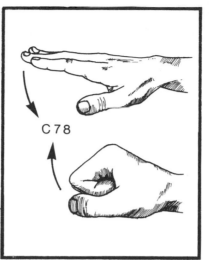

6. *Myotomes* (4) Both flexion and extension of the fingers are controlled by C7, 8.

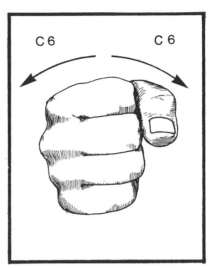

7. *Myotomes* (5) In the case of pronation and supination, a single spinal segment is involved, namely C6.

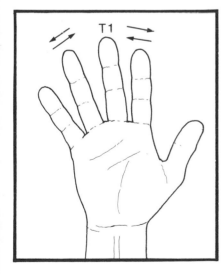

8. *Myotomes* (6) Again, a single segment, namely T1, is involved in producing abduction and adduction of the fingers ('small muscles of the hand').

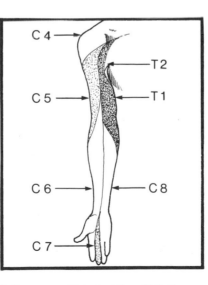

9. *Dermatomes* Note that the middle finger is supplied by C7, and that there is a regular sequence of sensory distribution round the pre-axial line of the arm.

10. *Plexus lesions* (1) *In Erb's Palsy* (upper obstetrical palsy) the wrist is flexed and pronated and the fingers flexed. The elbow is extended (waiter's tip deformity). The nerve to rhomboids and the long thoracic nerve are usually spared.

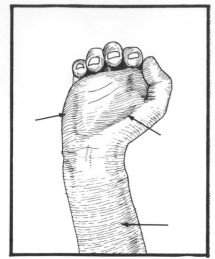

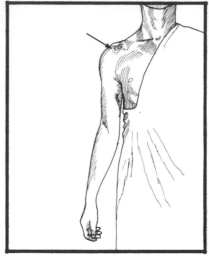

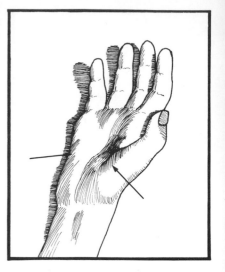

11. *Plexus lesions* (2) In *Klumpke's Paralysis* the small (intrinsic) muscles including the hypothenar and thenar groups are wasted and there is a claw hand deformity. There is sensory loss on the medial side of the forearm and wrist. In many cases there is an associated Horner syndrome.

12. *Plexus lesions* (3) *Traumatic traction lesions* (e.g., from motor-cycle accidents) may be accompanied by tell-tale bruising of the neck and shoulder where it has been depressed. In the more severe cases the anaesthetic limb hangs flaily at the side. The level of the lesion, and hence the prognosis or need for exploration may be assessed by clinical examination and myelography (see 1); sensory nerve conduction and electro-myographic studies may also be helpful.

13. *Plexus lesions* (4) *The T1 root* may be involved in spondylosis, Klumpke's Paralysis, cervical rib, neurofibromatosis, apical carcinoma, and metastases. There is wasting of the small muscles (including the thenar group) in the hand, but the sensory loss is entirely medial.

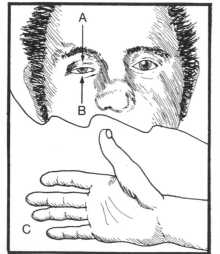

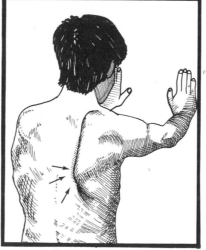

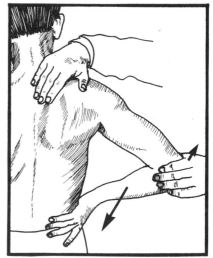

14. *Plexus lesions* (5) *Horner's Syndrome* occurs when the T1 root is involved close to the canal, with (A) pseudo-ptosis (B) smallness of the pupil on the affected side (C) dryness of the hand from absence of sweating.

15. *Nerve to Serratus Anterior* (C567). This nerve may be damaged by traction while lifting heavy weights. It usually causes little disability apart from winging of the scapula, which may be demonstrated by asking the patient to lean with both hands against a wall.

16. *Nerve to Rhomboids* (C5) Absence of rhomboid activity is indicative of a lesion proximal to the formation of the upper trunk of the plexus—i.e. a proximal C5 root lesion. Ask the patient to place the hand on the hip and to resist the elbow being pushed forwards. Feel for contraction in the muscle.

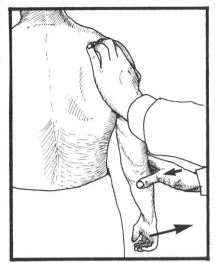

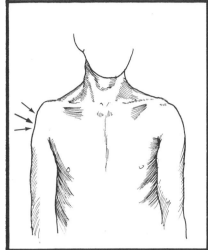

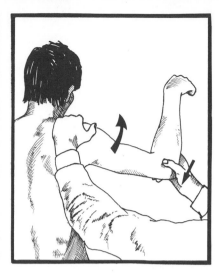

17. *Nerve to Supraspinatus* C56 Feel for contraction above the spine of the scapula as the patient abducts against resistance. Absence of contraction in the presence of intact rhomboids suggests an upper trunk lesion.

18. *Axillary Nerve.* C56 (1) This nerve is most commonly damaged during shoulder dislocations and displaced humeral neck fractures. Spontaneous recovery usually occurs. Flattening over the lateral aspect of the shoulder develops when muscle wasting is at its height.

19. *Axillary Nerve* (2) Ask the patient to attempt to move the arm from the side (pain permitting) while you resist any movement. Look for and feel for deltoid contraction. This is often difficult to assess, and the sides should be compared.

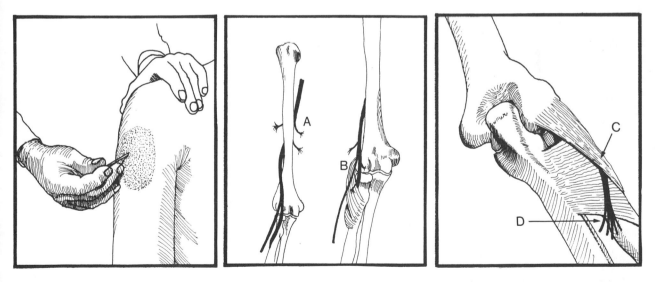

20. *Axillary Nerve* (3) Look for loss of sensation over the 'regimental badge' area of the shoulder, the exclusive distribution of the nerve.

21. *Radial Nerve:* (Posterior cord) C5678 (T1). *Motor distribution:* (A) In the upper arm triceps. (B) In the front of the elbow the radial and its post interosseous branch supply extensor carpi radialis longus, extensor carpi radialis brevis, brachioradialis, and part of supinator.

22. *Radial Nerve:* (Motor ctd) (C) In the supinator tunnel it supplies the rest of supinator. (D) On leaving supinator below the elbow it supplies extensor digitorum communis, extensor indicis, extensor digiti minimi, extensor carpi ulnaris, abductor pollicis longus, extensors pollicis longus and brevis.

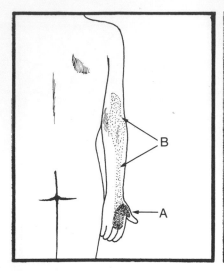

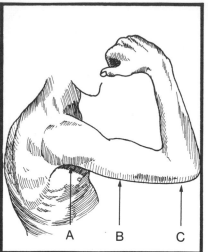

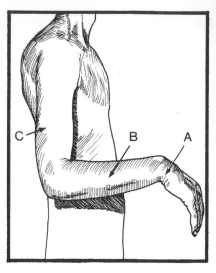

23. *Radial Nerve: Sensory distribution:* (A) The terminal part supplies the radial side of the back of the hand. (B) The posterior cutaneous branch of the radial, given off in the upper arm, supplies a variable area on the back of the arm and forearm.

24. *Radial Nerve: Common sites affected:* (A) In the axilla (e.g. from local pressure from crutches or the back of a chair in the so-called 'Saturday night' palsy), (B) mid-humerus (fracture and tourniquet palsy), (C) at and below the elbow (e.g. after dislocations of the elbow, Monteggia fractures, ganglions, surgical damage, etc.).

25. *Radial Nerve Examination* (1) (A) Is there an obvious drop wrist? (B) Is there wasting of the forearm muscles? (C) Is there wasting of the triceps, suggesting a high lesion?

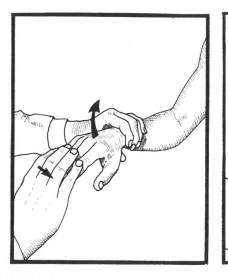

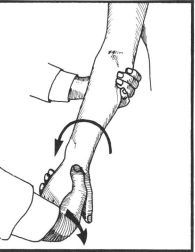

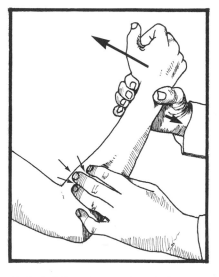

26. *Radial Nerve Examination* (2) Test the extensors of the wrist and fingers. The elbow should be flexed and the forearm pronated.

27. *Radial Nerve Examination* (3) Test the supinator. The elbow must be extended to counter the supinating action of biceps. Loss of supination suggests a lesion proximal to the exit of the supinator tunnel.

28. *Radial Nerve Examination* (4) Test brachio-radialis. Ask the patient to flex the elbow, in the mid-pronation position, against resistance. Feel and look for contraction in the muscle. Loss of contraction suggests a lesion above the supinator tunnel.

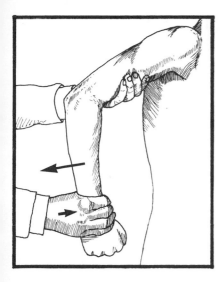

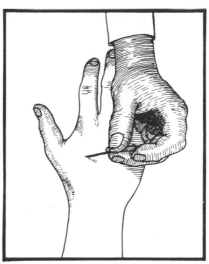

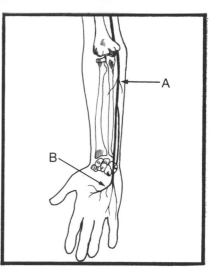

29. *Radial Nerve Examination* (5) Test the triceps. Extend the shoulder, and ask the patient to extend the elbow against gravity and then resistance. Weakness of triceps suggests a lesion at mid-humeral level, or an incomplete high lesion. Loss suggests a high, plexus lesion.

30. *Radial Nerve Examination* (6) Test for loss of sensation in the areas supplied by the nerve (see 23).

31. *Ulnar Nerve*: (Medial cord) C8T1: *Motor distribution:* (A) In the forearm, flexor carpi ulnaris and half of flexor digitorum profundus. (B) In the hand, the hypothenar muscles, the interossei, the two medial lumbricals and adductor pollicis.

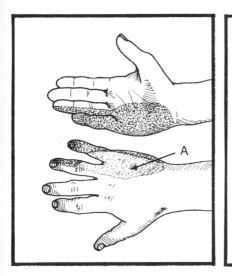

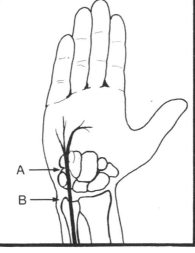

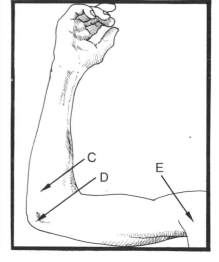

32. *Ulnar Nerve: Sensory distribution:* note that there are variations in the areas supplied by the median and ulnar nerves in the hand (the common distribution is shown). The branch supplying the dorsum (A) arises in the forearm. Loss here indicates a lesion *proximal to the wrist*.

33. *Ulnar Nerve: Common sites affected:* (A) In the ulnar tunnel, in the ulnar tunnel syndrome (e.g. from a ganglion). The most distal lesions affect the deep palmar nerve, and are entirely motor. (B) At the wrist, especially from lacerations, occupational trauma, and ganglions.

34. *Ulnar Nerve: Common sites ctd:* (C) Distal to the elbow, by compression between the two heads of flexor carpi ulnaris. (D) At the medial epicondyle (e.g. in cubitus valgus and in ulnar neuritis from osteo-arthritis and other causes), (E) in the brachial plexus, from trauma and other lesions.

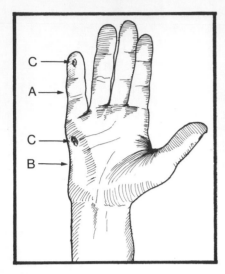

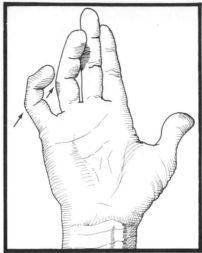

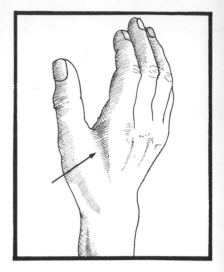

35. *Ulnar Nerve Examination* (1) Note the presence of (A) abduction of the little finger, (B) hypothenar wasting, (C) ulceration of the skin, brittleness of the nails and any other trophic changes.

36. *Ulnar Nerve Examination* (2) Note if there is an ulnar claw hand, with flexion of the ring and little fingers at the proximal I.P. joints. If the distal I.P. joints are flexed as well, this suggests that the flexor digitorum profundus is intact, and the lesion is distally placed; i.e. paradoxically, deformity of the hand is *less* marked in lesions proximal to the wrist where there is *more* motor involvement.

37. *Ulnar Nerve Examination* (3) Note the presence of any interosseous muscle wasting. The first dorsal interosseous is almost always the earliest to become noticeably affected, and the hollowing of the skin on the dorsal aspect of the first web space is often most striking.

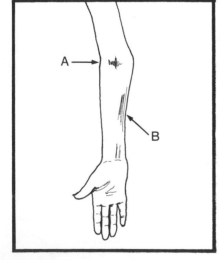

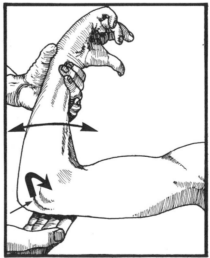

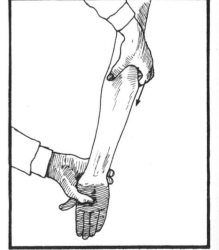

38. *Ulnar Nerve Examination* (4) Note (a) if there is any cubitus valgus or varus deformity suggesting an old injury such as a supracondylar fracture (of significance in tardy ulnar nerve palsy). (b) Wasting of muscle on the medial side of the forearm, confirming a lesion proximal to the wrist. Compare the sides.

39. *Ulnar Nerve Examination* (5) Flex and extend the elbow, looking for abnormal mobility in the nerve at the medial side of the joint. If the nerve is seen to snap over the medial epicondyle, a traumatic ulnar neuritis may be diagnosed with reasonable confidence.

40. *Ulnar Nerve Examination* (6) Roll the nerve under the fingers above the medial epicondyle and follow it distally until it disappears about 4 cm beyond the epicondyle under flex. carp. ulnaris. Note tenderness, thickening, or production of paraesthesiae.

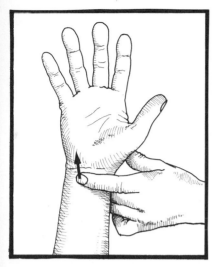

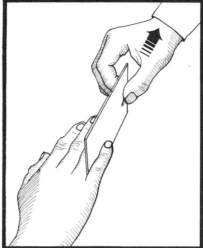

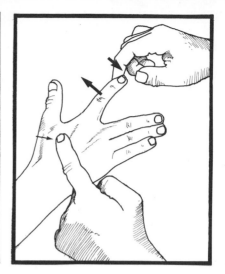

41. *Ulnar Nerve Examination* (7) Palpate the region of the nerve just lateral to flexor carpi ulnaris at the wrist, and follow it down to the ulnar tunnel region of the hand, again looking for undue tenderness and paraesthesiae.

42. *Ulnar Nerve* (8) *Interossei.* Ask the patient to hold a sheet of paper between the ring and little fingers. The fingers *must* be fully extended. Withdraw the paper, and note the resistance offered. In a complete palsy, the patient will be unable to grip the paper.

43. *Ulnar Nerve* (9) *First dorsal interosseous.* Place the palm face down and ask the patient to resist while you attempt to adduct the index. Look and feel for contraction in the first dorsal interosseous.

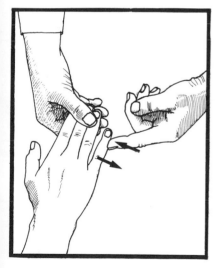

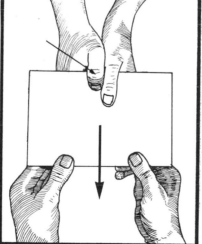

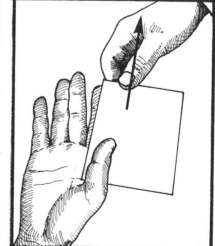

44. *Ulnar Nerve* (10) *Abductor digiti minimi:* Ask the patient to resist as you adduct the extended little finger with your index. Note the resistance offered, and compare the sides.

45. *Ulnar Nerve* (11) *Adductor pollicis:* Ask the patient to grasp a sheet of paper between the thumbs and sides of the index fingers while you attempt to withdraw it. If the adductor of the thumb is paralysed, the thumb will flex at the interphalangeal joint (Froment's test).

46. *Ulnar Nerve* (12) *Adductor pollicis:* Alternatively, test the patient's ability to grasp a sheet of paper between the thumb and the anterior aspect of the index metacarpal.

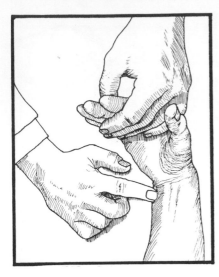

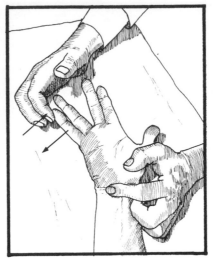

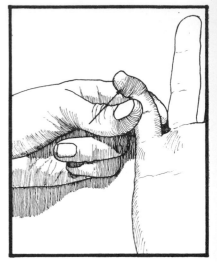

47. *Ulnar Nerve* (13) *Flexor carpi ulnaris* (1) Ask the patient to resist while you attempt to extend the flexed wrist. Feel for contraction of the tendon at the wrist.

48. *Ulnar Nerve* (14) *Flexor carpi ulnaris* (2) Place the hand on a flat surface and ask the patient to resist while you attempt to adduct the little finger. Again feel for contraction in the tendon. Loss of activity indicates a lesion proximal to the wrist.

49. *Ulnar Nerve* (15) *Flexor digitorum profundus:* Support the middle phalanx of the little finger and ask the patient to flex the distal joint. Apply counter pressure to the finger tip and note the resistance. Loss of power indicates a lesion near the elbow or above.

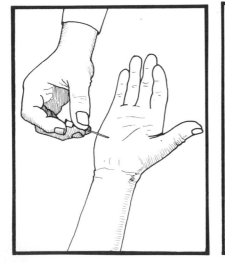

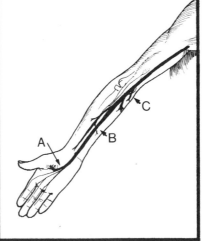

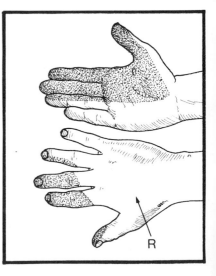

50. *Ulnar Nerve* (16) *Sensation.* Test for disturbance of pin-prick sensation in the area supplied by the nerve. Note loss on the dorsum indicates a lesion proximal to the wrist.

51. *Median Nerve* (Lat. and medial cords) C(5)678T1: *Motor distribution:* (A) Hand: Thenar muscles, lateral 2 lumbricals. (B) Forearm: flexor pollicis longus, half of flexor dig. profundus, pronator quadratus. (C) Near elbow: flexor digitorum sublimis, flexor carpi radialis, pronator teres.

52. *Median Nerve: Sensory distribution:* Note that there is considerable variation in the relative areas supplied by the median and ulnar nerves. Note also that the lateral side of the posterior aspect of the hand is supplied by the terminal part of the radial nerve (R). (The commonest pattern is shown.)

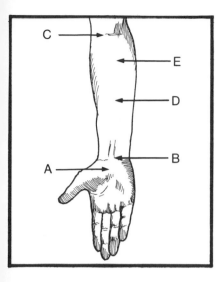

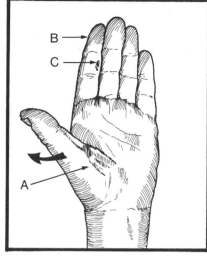

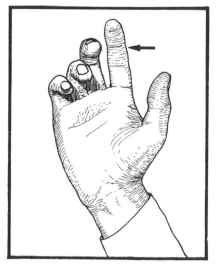

53. *Median Nerve: Common sites affected:*
(A) Carpal tunnel (e.g. carpal tunnel syndrome and carpal dislocations). (B) At the wrist (e.g. following wounds). (C) At elbow (e.g. after elbow dislocation in children). (D) In forearm (anterior interosseous nerve) e.g. after forearm fractures. (E) At level of pronator teres in the pronator teres nerve entrapement syndrome.

54. *Median Nerve: Examination:* Note (A) thenar wasting. In long standing cases the thumb may come to lie in the plane of the palm (Simian thumb). (B) Atrophy of the pulp of the index, cracking of nails and other trophic changes. (C) Cigarette burns and other signs of sensory loss.

55. *Median Nerve: Examination* (2): In lesions of the anterior interosseous branch or the median at or above the elbow, there may be wasting of the lateral aspect of the forearm, and the index is held in a position of extension (Benediction attitude).

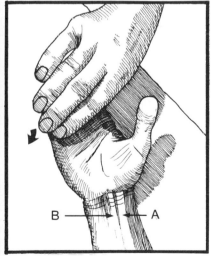

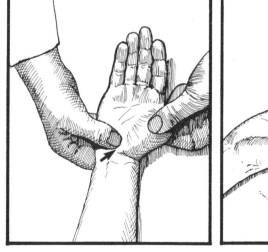

56. *Median Nerve: Examination* (3): First locate the position of the nerve. Attempt to extend the flexed wrist; palpate if necessary. The nerve lies between (A) flexor carpi radialis longus and (B) palmaris longus. (Or medial to flex. carpi. rad. longus if the latter is absent.)

57. *Median Nerve: Examination* (4): Look for tenderness on firm pressure over the nerve at the wrist and carpal tunnel. If the carpal tunnel syndrome is suspected, carry out the tapping, stretch and other tests detailed in the wrist section (Wrist 34–41).

58. *Medial Nerve: Examination* (5): *Abductor pollicis brevis* (1) This muscle is invariably and exclusively supplied by the median. To test, place the hand on a flat surface and hold your index above the palm.

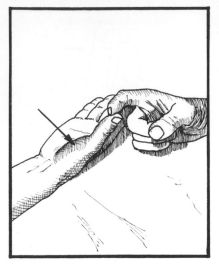

59. *Median Nerve: Examination* (6):
Abductor pollicis brevis (2) Ask the patient
to raise his thumb to touch the finger.
Look for contraction in the muscle.

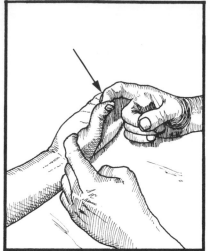

60. *Median Nerve: Examination* (7):
Abductor pollicis brevis (3) Ask the patient
to resist while you force it back. Note the
resistance offered; palpate the muscle to
confirm tone and bulk; compare the sides.

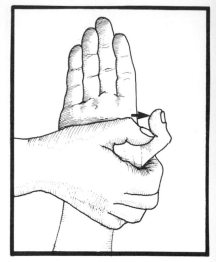

61. *Median Nerve: Examination* (8): Test
power in *flexor pollicis longus*, and *flexor
digitorum profundus* to the index. Loss of
power indicates a lesion above the wrist,
either of the anterior interosseous nerve, or
of the median nerve above the level of that
branch.

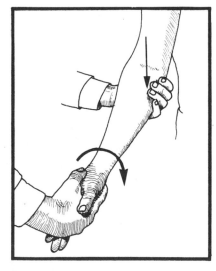

62. *Median Nerve: Examination* (9):
Pronator teres: Extend the elbow and feel
for contraction in the muscle as the patient
attempts to pronate the arm against
resistance. Loss indicates a high lesion of
the nerve, in the upper elbow region or
more proximal. Accompanying pain and
tenderness over the pronator teres is found
in the pronator teres entrapement
syndrome.

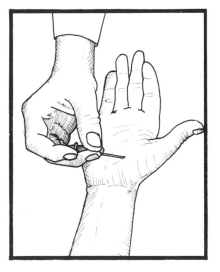

63. *Median Nerve: Examination* (10): Look
for impairment of sensation to pin prick in
the distribution of the nerve.

64. *Assessment of Motor Power:* Where
there is some loss of muscle power in a
limb, it is important to make accurate
records so that any improvement or
deterioration can be detected at a later
examination.

Either the power of individual muscles or
of specific movements (e.g. flexion and
extension of the elbow) should be
tabulated. The M.R.C. grading is
recommended:

0 = No active contraction can be detected.

1 = A flicker of muscle contraction can be
seen or found by palpation over the
muscle, but the activity is insufficient to
cause any joint movement.

2 = Contraction is very weak, but can just
produce movement so long as the weight
of the part can be countered by careful
positioning of the limb.

3 = Contraction is still very weak, but can
produce movement against gravitational
resistance (e.g. the quadriceps being able to
extend the knee with the patient in a
sitting position).

4 = Strength is not full, but can produce
movement against gravity and added
resistance.

5 = Normal power is present. (Compare
one side with the other.)

2 The Cervical Spine

Cervical spondylosis (cervical osteo-arthrosis: osteo-arthritis of the cervical spine)

Cervical spondylosis is easily the most common condition affecting the neck. Degenerative changes appear early in life in the cervical spine, often during the third decade. The disc space between the 5th and 6th cervical vertebrae is most frequently involved. The earliest changes are confined to the disc, but the facet joints and the unco-vertebral joints (joints of Luschka) may soon become involved. There is inevitable restriction of movements at the affected level, but this is often impossible to detect clinically as it is masked by persisting mobility in the joints above and below. The condition may in fact never attract attention, but unfortunately in many cases symptoms do occur, sometimes being triggered off by minor trauma. Pain may be felt centrally in the neck, and may radiate to the occiput, giving rise to severe occipital headache which may be confused with migraine; pain may also radiate in a downward direction further than might be expected on anatomical grounds, to the region of the lower scapulae. Often there is pain at the side of the neck, quite sharply localised, or in the supraclavicular region. With nerve root involvement from arthritic changes in the facet or unco-vertebral joints, there may be radiation of pain into the shoulders, arms and hands, with paraesthesiae and on rare occasions demonstrable neurological involvement; this may include absent arm reflexes, muscle weakness, and sensory impairment. The cervical cord may be compressed by a central disc protrusion or from osteophytes arising from the posterior aspects of the vertebral bodies, giving rise to long tract signs and disturbance of gait. Vertebral artery involvement by osteophytic outgrowth may cause drop attacks precipitated by extension of the neck. Osteophytes arising from the anterior vertebral margins may sometimes by their size give rise to dysphagia.

In the 20 to 35 age group, often before there is any radiological evidence of arthritic change in the spine, a sudden movement of the neck may produce severe neck and arm pain accompanied by striking protective muscle spasm and limitation of cervical movements. In some cases these symptoms are produced by an acute disc prolapse similar to those occurring more familiarly in the lumbar region. In others, with identical symptoms, myelography may be quite negative, and some disturbance of the facet joints or related structures of often thought responsible.

The mainstay of treatment in spondylosis is the judicious use of a cervical collar and the prescription of analgesics. If root symptoms are prominent, intermittent or continuous cervical traction is often employed. Manipulation of the cervical spine, especially in the younger age groups with no neurological involvement, is sometimes advocated. Severe, protracted symptoms may be investigated further by myelography. If a positive lesion is demonstrated, exploration may be carried out; if not, a local cervical fusion may sometimes be advised.

Cervical rib syndrome

Symptoms in the arm from involvement of the brachial plexus and axillary artery by a cervical rib is a definite but rare occurrence. Slightly more commonly, the same structures may be kinked by fibrous bands or abnormalities in the scalene attachments at the root of the neck. Paraesthesiae in the hand are severe, and there may be hypothenar and less commonly thenar wasting. There is sometimes sympathetic disturbance with increased sweating of the hand. The radial pulse may be absent, and other signs of vascular impairment may be present. Complete vascular occlusion, sometimes accompanied by thrombosis and emboli, may lead to gangrene of the finger tips. In some cases symptoms may be precipitated by loss of tone in the shoulder girdle, with drooping of the shoulders; in such cases, physiotherapy is often successful in restoring tone to the affected muscles and relieving symptoms. When vascular involvement predominates, arteriography and exploration may be required.

Whiplash and extension injuries of the neck

Whiplash injuries are now a common cause of persistent cervical symptoms. A true whiplash injury occurs classically when as a result of a rear impact, a stationary or slowly moving vehicle strikes another vehicle or object in front. Because of the inertial mass of the head of the car occupant, there is rapid extension of the cervical spine followed by flexion. In the partial whiplash injury, the main element is extension of the neck; this also commonly occurs as a result of a rear impact, but in this case the vehicle in which the occupant is travelling comes to rest more gradually without striking anything ahead. In the majority of cases the radiographs show normal alignment of the cervical vertebrae but occasionally small avulsion fractures of the anterior margins of the vertebral bodies give evidence of the forcible extension of the spine. In some cases there are minor fractures involving the unco-vertebral joints. Where there are spondylotic changes which interfere with the dissipation of the forces involved because of localised areas of rigidity in the spine, there may be avulsion of anterior osteophytes. The flexion element may sometimes produce wedge compression fractures of the vertebral bodies or avulsion fractures of the spinous processes. These injuries produce symptoms of all degrees of severity. There is always pain and stiffness in the neck, with often neurological disturbance involving the upper and sometimes the lower limbs. Even minor symptoms may be most protracted, lasting often 18 months or longer. In some cases, disability is permanent. Cervical collar supports, local heat and analgesics are usually advised.

Severe extension injuries occur in falls (often downstairs) when the neck is forcibly extended as the head strikes the ground. There is often tell-tale bruising of the forehead. In car accidents an unbelted occupant may suffer severe extension of the neck in the early phases of deceleration when the forehead strikes the roof and ricochets backwards. In both sets of circumstances the head injury may attract prior attention, but the possibility of these injuries must not be overlooked. Cervical spondylosis again has a deleterious localising effect on the forces involved, and the neurological disturbance may be profound. In some cases thrombosis extends from the area of local cord involvement, so that there may be a deteriorating and sometimes fatal neurological outcome.

Rheumatoid arthritis in the cervical spine

Rheumatoid arthritis often involves the neck, and often in a patchy fashion so that additional stresses are thrown on the remaining mobile elements. With the ligamentous stretching that often accompanies rheumatoid arthritis there may be progressive subluxation of the cervical spine particularly at the atlanto-axial and mid-cervical levels. As this progresses, pain and stiffness in the neck become accompanied by root and cord symptoms. In the case of atlanto-axial subluxations, there may be severe occipital headache. The gait tends to become ataxic and there is progressive paralysis, often with bladder involvement.

These lesions are usually treated by local cervical fusion if the patient's general condition will allow.

Neoplasms in the cervical region

Tumours of the cervical spine are rare, secondary deposits however being the most common. They may cause vertebral body erosion or collapse, affect issuing nerve roots, or give rise to cord involvement. Of the primary tumours in this region sarcoma and multiple myeloma are the most common. Primary involvement of the cord may arise with meningiomas and intradural neurofibromata, which may also affect isolated nerve roots.

Infections

Tuberculosis of the cervical spine occurs most commonly in children, and may produce widespread bone destruction with collapse and cord involvement. Other infections are rare.

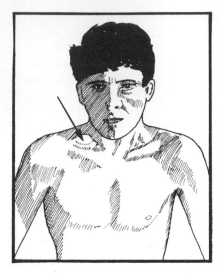

1. *Inspection* (1) Note any asymmetry in the supraclavicular fossae which will require separate investigation (e.g. Pancoast tumour).

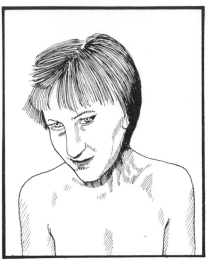

2. *Inspection* (2) Note the presence of torticollis which often results from protective spasm associated with trauma, tonsillar infection or vertebral body disease. In advanced infections and tumours the head may be supported by the hands. If the patient is an infant, note if a sternomastoid tumour is present.

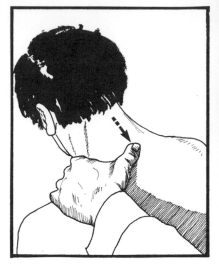

3. *Palpation* (1) Begin by looking for tenderness in the midline from the occiput downwards. Tenderness localised to one space is common in cervical spondylosis and in the very much rarer infections of the cervical spine.

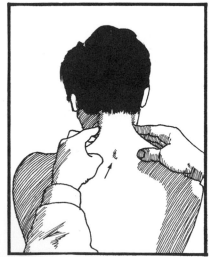

4. *Palpation* (2) Now palpate the lateral aspects of the vertebrae looking for masses and tenderness. Note that the most prominent spinous process is that of T1, and *not* the vertebra prominens, C7.

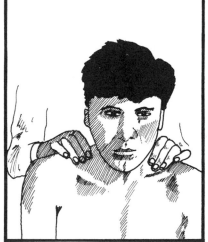

5. *Palpation* (3) Continue palpation into the supraclavicular fossae, looking particularly for the prominence of a cervical rib with local tenderness; look also for tumour masses and enlarged cervical lymph nodes.

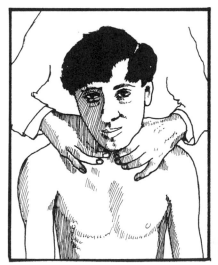

6. *Palpation* (4) Complete palpation of the neck by examining the anterior structures including the thyroid gland.

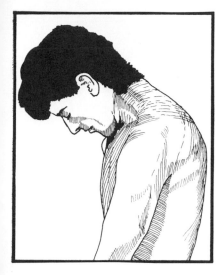

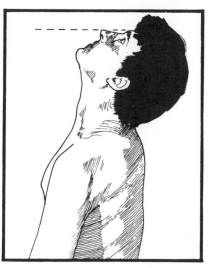

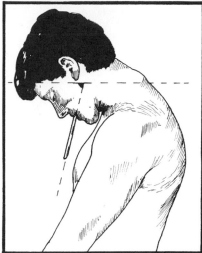

7. *Movements* (1) *Flexion.* Ask the patient to bend the head forwards. Normally the chin can be brought down to touch the region of the sterno-clavicular joints. The chin-chest distance may be measured for record purposes.

8. *Movements* (2) *Extension.* Ask the patient to tilt the head backwards. The patient should be seated and erect. The plane of nose and forehead should normally be nearly horizontal but guard against contributory thoracic and lumbar spine movements.

9. *Movements* (3) Recording motion in the cervical spine with any accuracy is difficult, but may be attempted using a goniometer. The patient should hold a spatula in the clenched teeth, and this may be used as a pointer. Ask the patient to flex the head forwards.

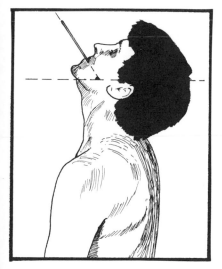

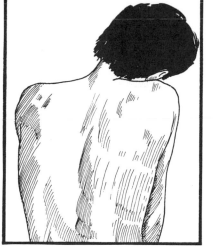

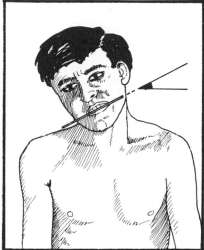

10. *Movements* (4) Now ask the patient to extend the head. The range between flexion and extension can then be measured.
Normal range = 130°
Of the total range of flexion and extension, about a fifth occurs in the atlanto-axial and atlanto-occipital joints.

11. *Movements* (5) *Lateral flexion.* Ask the patient to tilt his head onto his right shoulder. Lateral flexion with slight shoulder shrugging will allow the ear to touch the shoulder. Repeat on the other side and note any difference.

12. *Movements* (6) *Lateral flexion.* For greater accuracy, a spatula clenched in the teeth may again be used as a pointer.
Normal range = 45°
About a fifth of this movement occurs at the atlanto-axial and atlanto-occipital joints. Loss is common in cervical spondylosis.

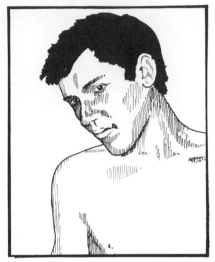

13. *Movements* (7) If lateral flexion cannot be carried out without forward flexion, this is indicative of involvement of the atlanto-axial and atlanto-occipital joints.

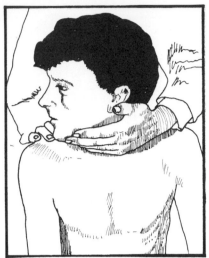

14. *Movements* (8) *Rotation* (1) Ask the patient to look over the shoulder. The movement may be encouraged with one hand, and movement of the shoulder restrained with the other. Normally the chin just falls short of the plane of the shoulders.

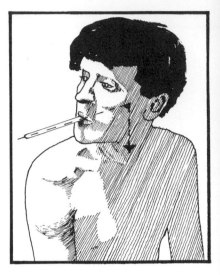

15. *Movements* (9) *Rotation* (2) Again a spatula may be used as a pointer for measurement.
Normal range = 80° to either side
About a third of this occurs in the first two cervical joints. Rotation is usually restricted and painful in cervical spondylosis.

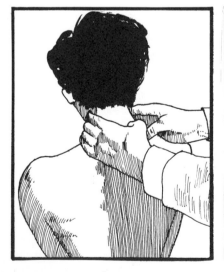

16. *Crepitations.* Spread the hands on each side of the neck and ask the patient to flex and extend the spine. Facet joint crepitation is normally detectable in this fashion in cervical spondylosis.

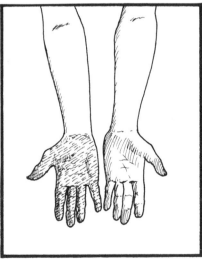

17. *Cervical rib* (1) Look for evidence of ischaemia in one hand (e.g. coldness, discolouration, trophic changes). Bilateral changes are more in favour of Raynaud's disease.

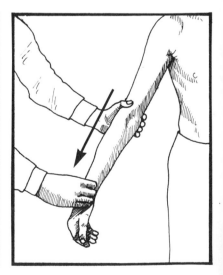

18. *Cervical rib* (2) Palpate the radial pulse and apply traction to the arm.
Obliteration of the pulse is not diagnostic, but when the test reveals no change when repeated on the other side it is suggestive.

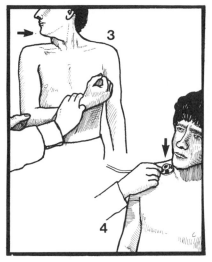

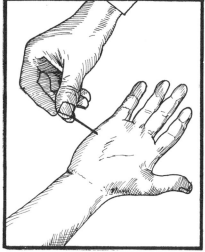

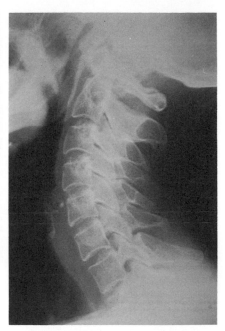

19. *Cervical rib* (3) Ask the patient to turn his head towards the affected side and to take a deep breath (and hold it). If the radial pulse is obliterated (from scalenus anterior obstruction) this is suggestive of the syndrome. (4) Auscultate over the subclavian artery. A murmur is suggestive of a mechanical obstruction, but repeat on the other side.

20. *Neurological examination:* Examination of the segmental distributions in the upper limbs is essential. In addition, the plantar responses should be checked for evidence of long tract involvement.

21. *Radiographs* (1) *Lateral:* The standard projections are the lateral, and A-P views of the lower and upper cervical vertebrae.

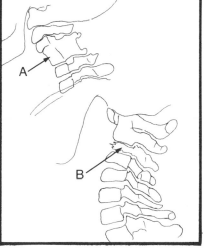

22. *Radiographs* (2) Begins your study of the lateral projection by noting the cervical curve which is normally slightly convex anteriorly: (A) normal, regular curve, (B) loss of curvature (which may be a positional error or suggest protective spasm), (C) kinking (from a local lesion, e.g. subluxation).

23. *Radiographs* (3) Now look at the general shape of the bodies of the vertebrae, comparing one with another. Note for example, (A) congenital vertebral fusion, (B) vertebral collapse from tuberculosis, tumour or fracture.

24. *Radiographs* (4) Note the relationship of each vertebra to the one above and below. It is helpful to trace the posterior margins of the bodies. Displacement occurs in dislocations, and may be small when the facet joints on one side only are involved.

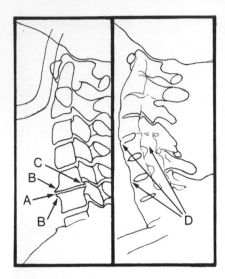

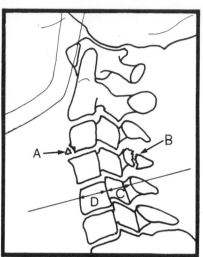

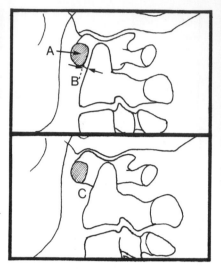

25. *Radiographs* (5) Look at the disc spaces and the related margins of the vertebrae. Note (A) disc space narrowing, (B) anterior lipping, (C) posterior lipping (all typical of cervical spondylosis). Note any evidence of fusion (D) typical of ankylosing spondylitis.

26. *Radiographs* (6) Note the presence (A) of an osteophyte or marginal fracture, suggestive of an extension injury of the neck, (B) fracture of a spinous process, suggestive of a flexion injury of the cervical spine. Syringomyelia (which can produce pain in the head, neck and limbs) may cause vertebral body erosions and dilatation of the canal. The diameter of the canal at C5(C) should not exceed the vertebral body diameter (D) by more than 6 mm.

27. *Radiographs* (7) (A) Note that the anterior arch of the atlas lies in front of the lower cervical vertebrae. (B) The distance between the arch and the axis is normally 1–4 mm. A greater distance (C) suggests rupture or laxity of the transverse ligament (e.g. from trauma, rheumatoid arthritis or infection).

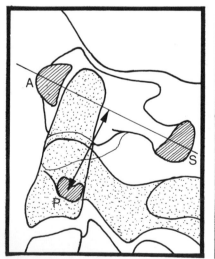

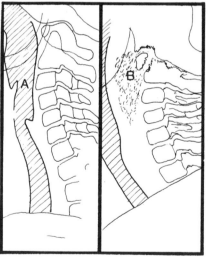

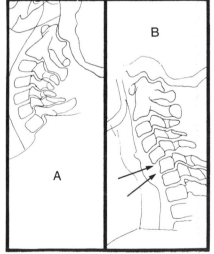

28. *Radiographs* (8) Upward (cranial) migration of the odontoid process is also commonly seen in rheumatoid arthritis. In the adult this may be assessed by noting the distance between the pedicle (P) of C2 (shown stippled) and a line connecting the spinous process (S) with the arch (A) of C1. If this is less than 11.5 mm, upward migration is considered to be present.

29. *Radiographs* (9) Note the pharyngeal shadow which normally lies fairly close to the bodies of the vertebrae as at (A). Displacement suggests a retro-pharyngeal mass, e.g. (B) sub-occipital tuberculosis with abscess. Other causes include haematoma and tumour.

30. *Radiographs* (10) Where instability is suspected, the lateral projection should be supervised with the neck (A) in extension, (B) in flexion. Any latent instability should be discernible by comparing these views. If doubt remains, intensifier screening of movement may help.

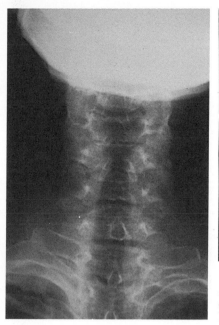

31. *Radiographs* (11) Normal A-P view of the lower cervical vertebrae.

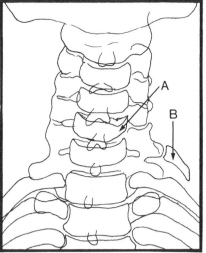

32. *Radiographs* (12) In the A-P view, interpretation is difficult due to the complexity of the superimposed structures. Note the shape of the vertebral bodies, observing (A) any lateral wedging, e.g. from fracture, tumour or infection. Note (B) the presence of any cervical rib.

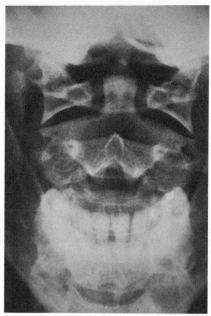

33. *Radiographs* (13) Normal A-P (through-the-mouth) view of C1–3.

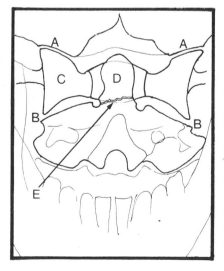

34. *Radiographs* (14) In the A-P view of C1–3, note (A) the atlanto-occipital joints, (B) the atlanto-axial joints, (C) the lateral masses of the atlas. Note any lack of symmetry in the alignment of the odontoid process (D) with the atlas, and look for any evidence of fracture (E).

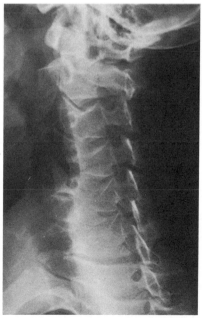

35. *Radiographs* (15) Normal oblique projection of the cervical spine (one of two).

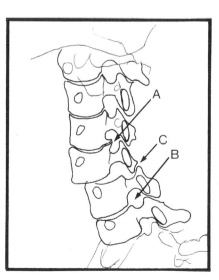

36. *Radiographs* (16) Right and left oblique projections are invaluable in demonstrating (A) localised lipping in the unco-vertebral joints (joints of Luschka) which may be encroaching the neural foramina (B). They may also show overlapping (locked) facet joints (C) in cervical subluxations.

3 The Shoulder

The commonest cause of shoulder pain is cervical spondylosis. Pain from irritation of nerve roots in the neck is referred to the shoulder in the same way as pain originating in the lumbar spine may be referred to the hip. There may on occasion be simultaneous pathology in both shoulder and neck, but differentiation is usually straightforward; in particular, restriction of movements of the shoulder with pain at the extremes points to the shoulder as the site of the principal pathology. Where symptoms are referred from the cervical spine, pain on movement, especially with a referred element, is more significant than restriction of movements.

'Frozen shoulder'

'Frozen shoulder' is a clinical syndrome which can probably be produced by a variety of pathological processes in the shoulder joint. These can seldom be differentiated and treatment is empirical. It is a condition affecting the middle-aged, in whose shoulder cuffs degenerative changes are occurring. The outstanding feature is limitation of movements in the shoulder. This restriction is often severe, with virtually no gleno-humeral movements possible, but in the milder cases rotation, especially internal rotation, is primarily affected. Restriction of movements is accompanied in most cases by pain, which is often severe and may disturb sleep. There is frequently a history of a minor trauma, which is usually presumed to produce some tearing of the degenerating shoulder cuff, thereby initiating the low grade prolonged inflammatory changes responsible for the symptoms. Radiographs of the shoulder are almost always normal. In some cases the condition is initiated by a period of immobilisation of the arm, not uncommonly as the result of the inadvised prolonged use of a sling after a Colles fracture. It is commoner on the left side, and in an appreciable number of cases there is a preceding episode of a silent or overt cardiac infarct. If untreated, pain subsides after many months, but permanent restriction of movements is common. The main aim of treatment is to improve the final range of movements in the shoulder, and graduated shoulder exercises are the mainstay of treatment. In some cases where pain is a particular problem, hydrocortisone injections into the shoulder cuff may be helpful. In a few cases, once the acute stage is well past, manipulation of the shoulder under general anaesthesia may be helpful in restoring movements in a stiff joint.

Shoulder cuff tears

The shoulder cuff may suffer a substantial tear as a result of sudden traction to the arm. This occurs most readily in the middle-aged where degenerative changes in the shoulder cuff have become established. Most commonly the supraspinatus region is involved, and the patient has difficulty in initiating abduction of the arm. In other cases a torn or inflamed shoulder cuff impinges on the acromion during abduction, giving rise to a painful arc of movement. Although the range of passive movements is not initially disturbed, limitation of rotation may supervene, so that many of these cases become ultimately indistinguishable from those suffering from frozen shoulder, and their treatment is essentially the same.

Calcifying supraspinatus tendinitis

Degenerative changes in the shoulder cuff may be accompanied by the local deposition of calcium salts. This process may continue without symptoms although radiographic changes are obvious. Sometimes, however, the calcified material may give rise to inflammatory changes in the subdeltoid bursa. Sudden, severe, incapacitating pain results; the shoulder is acutely tender, and often swollen and warm to the touch. Symptoms are relieved by the removal of the material by aspiration or curettage, but often local injections of hydrocortisone suffice. The joint is frequently so acutely tender that general anaesthesia is necessary for any attempted aspiration and injection of hydrocortisone.

O-A of the A-C joint

Arthritic changes in the A-C joint may give rise to prolonged pain associated with shoulder movements. There is usually an obvious prominence of the joint from arthritic lipping, with well localised tenderness. Conservative treatment with local heat and exercises may be helpful, but occasionally, in severe persistent cases, acromionectomy may be considered.

Recurrent dislocation of the shoulder

This condition is seen in the 20 to 40 age group. There is a history of previous frank dislocations of the shoulder in which the causal trauma has usually become progressively less severe. There is sometimes a history suggesting that the period of fixation after the initial injury was abbreviated. The shoulder is usually symptom-free between incidents. Surgical repair is usually advised if there have been four or more dislocations.

Infections round the shoulder

Staphylococcal osteitis of the proximal humerus is the commonest infection occurring near the shoulder in this country at present; nevertheless it is comparatively uncommon.

Tuberculosis of the shoulder is now rare. In the moist form, commonest in the first two decades of life, the shoulder is swollen, there is abundant pus production, and sinuses may form; the progress is comparatively rapid and destructive. In the dry form, caries sicca, an older age group is affected and the progress is slow with little destruction or pus formation; it is thought that many of the cases of caries sicca described in the past were in fact suffering from frozen shoulder.

Gonococcal arthritis of the shoulder. This infection is uncommon, but when it occurs there is moderate swelling of the joint and great pain which often seems out of keeping with the physical signs.

Miscellaneous conditions round the shoulder

A-C dislocation. The A-C joint may be disturbed as a result of a fall on the outstretched hand. If care is taken during examination a lesion of this joint will not be confused with one of the gleno-humeral joint. In major injuries, the conoid and trapezoid ligaments are torn and the clavicle is very unstable: surgical fixation of the clavicle to the coronoid is usually advised. In less severe cases, the A-C capsular ligaments only are torn; although the outer end of the clavicle becomes prominent, it follows the movement of the acromion and conservative treatment with a sling for several weeks is all that is required. These injuries are frequently missed as they often do not show in the routine recumbent radiographs of the shoulder.

Clavicle. Primary pathology in the clavicle is uncommon, but a cause of confusion is pathological fracture due to radio-necrosis years after treatment for breast carcinoma. The fracture may be preceded by pain for many months, and be mistaken for metastatic spread.

Scapula. Snapping scapula. A patient may complain of a grinding sensation arising from beneath the scapula. This is often due to a rib prominence, but in some cases may be caused by an exostosis arising from the deep surface of the scapula. When symptoms are persistant, excision of such as exostosis may give relief.

High scapula. There are several related congenital malformations affecting the neck and shoulder girdle. In the most minor cases one scapula may be a little smaller than the other and be more highly placed; in more severe cases one or both shoulders are highly situated, the scapulae are small, and there may be webs of skin running from the shoulder to the neck (Sprengel shoulder). In the Klippel Feil syndrome the neck is short and there are multiple anomalies of the cervical vertebrae; the scapulae are also highly situated.

Winged scapula. The patient complains of prominence of the scapula which is raised along its vertebral border from the chest wall. This is due to weakness of the serratus anterior. The cause may be primarily muscular (as in progressive muscular dystrophy) or follow traumatic paralysis of the long thoracic nerve. Active treatment is seldom necessary.

Ruptured biceps tendon. Rupture of the long head of biceps may occur spontaneously or as a result of a sudden muscular effort, usually in an elderly or middle-aged person in whom degenerative tendon changes are present. No treatment is usually required.

Sterno-clavicular joint. Dislocation of the S-C joint is comparatively uncommon; there is always a history of trauma, and the joint asymmetry is obvious if looked for. Good radiographs are often hard to obtain and their interpretation is difficult. The diagnosis should be made primarily on clinical grounds. Symptoms of pain on movement normally settle spontaneously, and only rarely is surgical repair required.

O-A and R-A. Osteo-arthritis of the gleno-humeral joint is rare and when it occurs is most frequently secondary to aseptic necrosis of the humeral head. This may be of idiopathic origin, follow high fractures of the humeral neck, or occur in caisson workers and deep sea divers.

Rheumatoid arthritis is more common, and the features are similar to those of the condition in other joints.

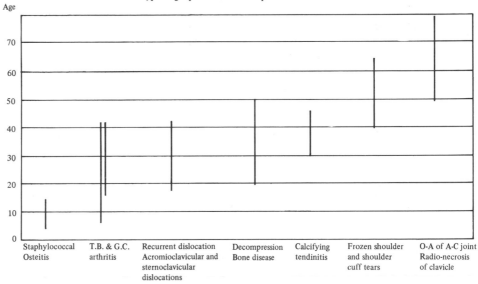

Typical Age Spread of the More Important Shoulder Conditions

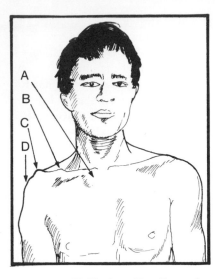

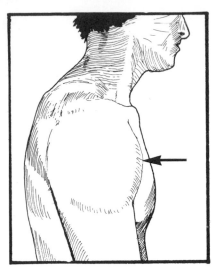

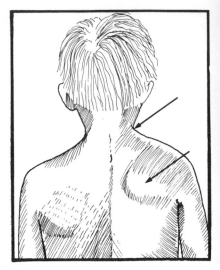

1. *Inspection* (1) *The front*. Note if any of the following are present: (A) Prominent sterno-clavicular joint (subluxation). (B) Deformity of clavicle (old fracture). (C) Prominent acromio-clavicular joint (subluxation or O-A). (D) Deltoid wasting (disuse or axillary nerve palsy).

2. *Inspection* (2) *The side*. Note if there is any swelling of the joint, suggesting infection or inflammatory reaction, from, for example, calcifying supraspinatus tendinitis, or from trauma.

3. *Inspection* (3) *From behind*. Are the scapulae normally shaped and situated, or small and high as in Sprengel shoulder and the Klippel-Feil syndrome? Is there webbing of the skin at the root of the neck, also typical of the latter? Is there winging of the scapula due to paralysis of serratus anterior (see *Shoulder* 33)?

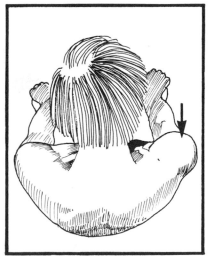

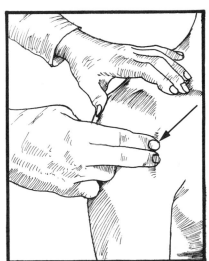

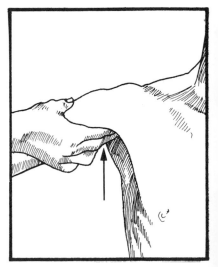

4. *Inspection* (4) *From above*. Again look for swelling of the shoulder, deformity of the clavicle, asymmetry of the supraclavicular fossae.

5. *Palpation* (1) Palpate the anterior and lateral aspects of the gleno-humeral joint. *Diffuse* tenderness is suggestive of infection or calcifying supraspinatus tendinitis.

6. *Palpation* (2) Continue the examination by palpating the upper humeral shaft and head via the axilla. Exostoses of the proximal humeral shaft are often readily palpable by this route.

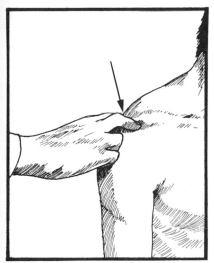

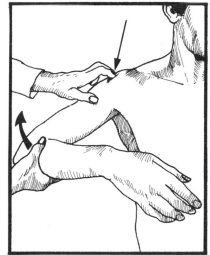

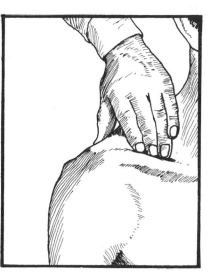

7. *Palpation* (3) Tenderness over the acromio-clavicular joint is found after recent dislocations, and in osteo-arthritis of the joint. In the latter, lipping is usually palpable, and crepitations may be detectable when the arm is abducted.

8. *Palpation* (4) Press below the acromion and abduct the arm. Sudden tenderness occurring during a portion of the arc of movement is found in tears and inflammatory lesions of the shoulder cuff.

9. *Palpation* (5) Palpate the length of the clavicle. Tenderness is found in sterno-clavicular dislocations and infections (particularly tuberculosis), tumours (rare), and radio-necrosis (usually after treatment for breast cancer). Radiological examination of the clavicle is essential if local tenderness is found.

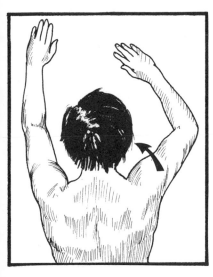

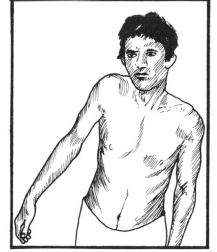

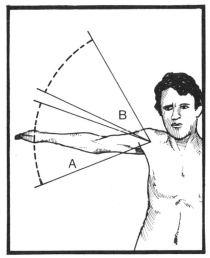

10. *Movements: Abduction* (1) Ask the patient to abduct both arms; observe the smoothness of the movement and the range achieved. A full, free and painless range is rare in the presence of any significant pathology in the shoulder region.

11. *Movements: Abduction* (2) Note any difficulty in initiating abduction. Difficulty in doing so is suggestive of a shoulder cuff (or supraspinatus tendon) tear.

12. *Movements: Abduction* (3) Note pain during abduction (which may have to be assisted). (A) Painful arc suggestive of shoulder cuff lesion (e.g. tear, degenerative changes). (B) Painful arc suggestive of osteo-arthritis of the acromio-clavicular joint.

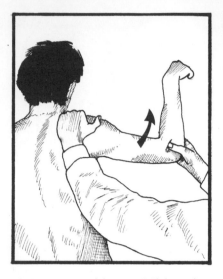

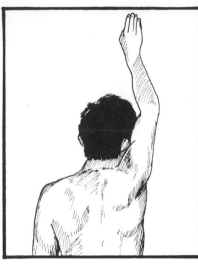

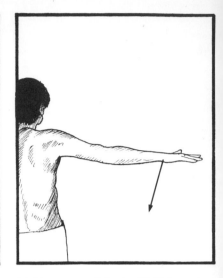

13. *Movements: Abduction* (4) If the patient cannot abduct the arm actively, attempt to do this passively, remembering to rotate the arm externally while doing so. A full range indicates an intact gleno-humeral joint.

14. *Movements: Abduction* (5) Ask the patient to hold the arm himself in the vertical position. If he can do so, deltoid and the axillary nerve are likely to be intact.

15. *Movements: Abduction* (6) If the patient has passed the last test, ask him to lower the arm to the side. Again note the presence of any painful arc of movement.

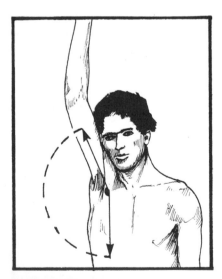

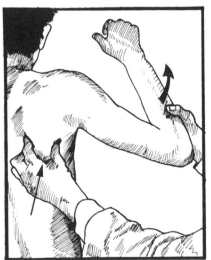

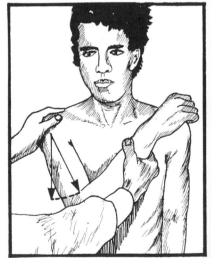

16. *Movements: Abduction* (7) Measure the range of abduction. In the normal shoulder, the arm can touch the ear with only slight tilting of the head. The shoulders have already been compared (10).
Normal range: 0–170°

17. *Movements: Abduction* (8) If both active and passive movements are restricted, fix the angle of the scapula with one hand, and try to abduct the arm with the other. Absence of movement indicates a fixed gleno-humeral joint, the previously noted movements having been entirely scapular.

18. *Movements: Abduction in extension:* Place one hand on the shoulder, and swing the arm, flexed at the elbow, across the chest.
Normal range: 0–50°

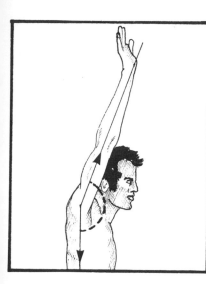

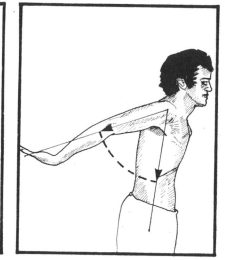

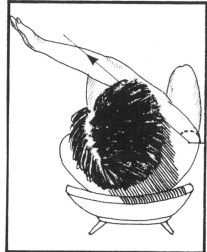

19. *Movements: Forward flexion:* Ask the patient to swing the arm forwards and lift it above his head. View the patient from the side.
Normal range: 0–165°

20. *Movements: Backwards extension:* Ask the patient to swing the arm directly backwards, again viewing and measuring from the side.
Normal range: 0–60°

21. *Movements: Horizontal flexion:* Occasionally measurement of this angle may be helpful, but it need not be routine. View the patient from above. The arm is moved forwards from a position of 90° abduction.
Normal range: 0–140°

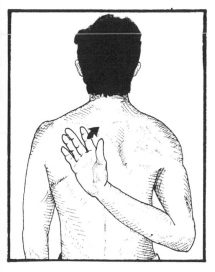

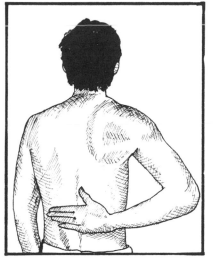

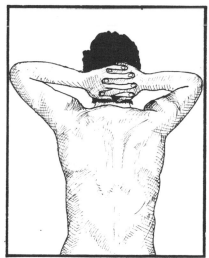

22. *Movements: Rotation screening tests* (1) Ask the patient to place the hand behind the opposite shoulder blade. This is a useful test of *internal rotation in extension.*

23. *Movements: Rotation screening* (2) With slight restriction, he will not be able to get the hand far up the back. With severe restriction, he will not be able to get the hand behind the back at all. This movement is commonly affected in frozen shoulder.

24. *Movements: Rotation screening* (3) Ask the patient to place both hands behind the head to screen *external rotation at 90° abduction.* Compare the two sides. Lack of success or restriction is common in frozen shoulder.

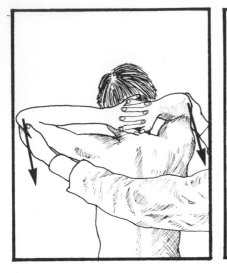

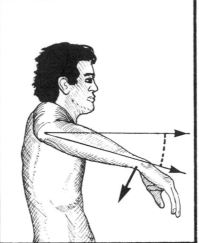

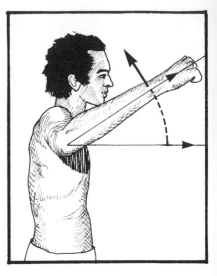

25. *Movements: Rotation screening* (4) Sometimes in the last test the patient gets the hand on the affected side behind the head, but in horizontal flexion. If so, gently pull both elbows backwards, noting any difference. (Pain and restriction common in frozen shoulder.)

26. *Movements: Internal rotation in abduction:* Abduct the shoulder to 90°, and flex the elbow to a right angle. Ask the patient to lower the forearm from the horizontal plane.
Normal range: 70°

27. *Movements: External rotation in abduction:* From the same starting position with the forearm parallel to the ground, ask the patient to raise the hand, keeping the shoulder in 90° abduction.
Normal range: 100°

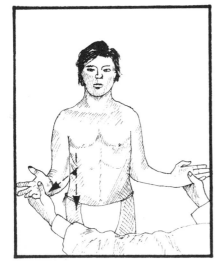

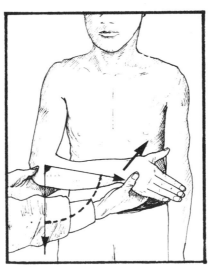

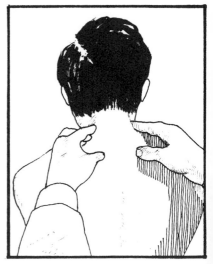

28. *Movements: External rotation in extension:* Place the elbows into the sides, and flex to 90°, with the hands facing forwards. Move the hands laterally, comparing one side with the other.
Normal range: 70°

29. *Movements: Internal rotation in extension:* Move the hand to the chest from the facing forward position. *Normal range: 70°. For clinical work, assessment of abduction and screening rotation should suffice (but record angular range of movements in all planes for monitoring progress and for medico-legal reports).*

30. *Cervical spine:* Always screen the cervical spine in examining a case of shoulder pain; this is doubly important if shoulder movements are found to be normal.

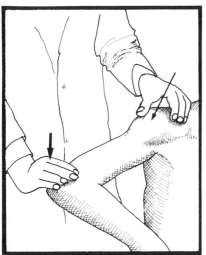 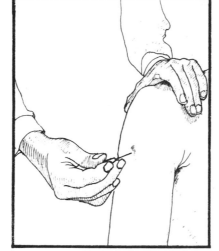 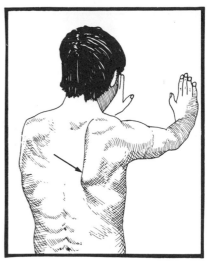

31. *Deltoid power:* Ask the patient to keep the arm elevated while you press down on the elbow. Look and feel for deltoid contraction. Note that deltoid palsy accompanies traction injuries of the axillary nerve (e.g. after dislocation of the shoulder).

32. *Axillary nerve:* Test for the presence of deltoid activity. Examine the 'regimental badge' area on the lateral aspect of the arm for sensory loss. Loss of sensation here is suggestive of axillary nerve palsy.

33. *Long thoracic nerve:* Where paralysis of serratus anterior is suspected, ask the patient to lean with both hands against a wall. Any tendency to winging of the scapula immediately becomes apparent.

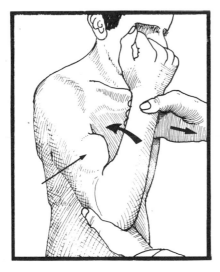 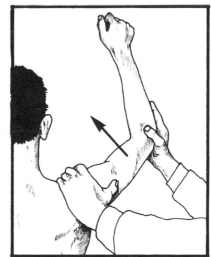

34. *Long head of biceps:* Support the patient's elbow with one hand. Grasp his wrist, and ask him to pull toward his shoulder, while you resist this movement. If the long tendon of biceps is ruptured, the belly of biceps will appear globular in shape. Compare sides.

35. *Crepitations:* Place one hand over the shoulder, with the middle finger lying along the acromio-clavicular joint. Abduct the arm with the other hand. Detect any crepitations coming from the shoulder, and locate their source (gleno-humeral or acromio-clavicular).

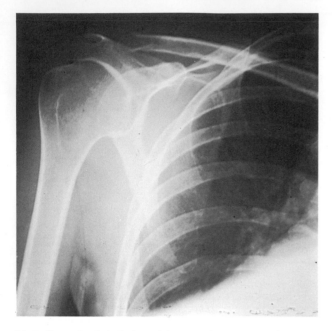

36. *Radiographs* (1) A-P view of the normal shoulder.

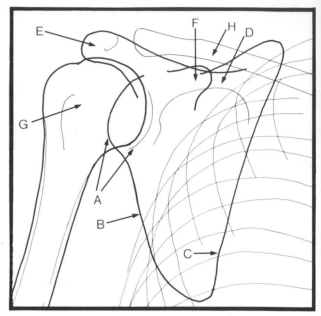

37. *Radiographs* (2) The standard shoulder projection is the A-P taken in recumbency. Examine the radiograph methodically by identifying (A) the glenoid, (B) the lateral border of the scapula, (C) the medial border, (D) its spine, (E) the acromion, (F) the coracoid. Note the relations of (G) the humeral head and (H) the clavicle to the glenoid and the acromion.

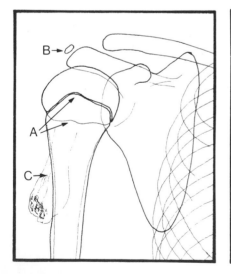

38. *Radiographs* (3) Do not mistake (A) the anterior and posterior margins of the epiphysis for fracture or (B) the acromial ossification centre for a loose body. Note (C) the typical appearance of a simple exostosis (ossifying chondroma) of epiphyseal plate origin.

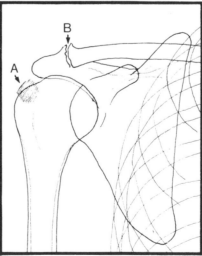

39. *Radiographs* (4) Calcification in the supraspinatus tendon in the upper part of the shoulder cuff has an amorphous appearance (A) and is characteristically situated. It may be symptom free. Note (B) arthritic changes in the acromio-clavicular joint.

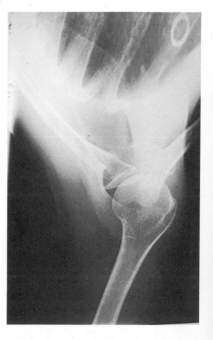

40. *Radiographs* (5) Normal axial lateral.

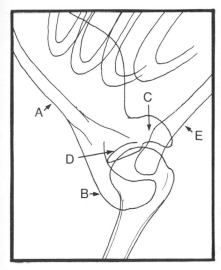

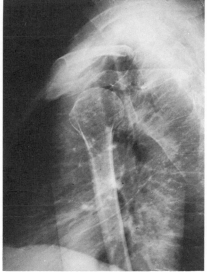

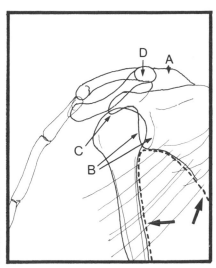

41. *Radiographs* (6) The axial lateral gives the most useful additional information, but is dependent on the patient being able to abduct the arm. It is very helpful in clarifying the relationships of the glenoid and humeral head. (A) Scapula spine, (B) acromion, (C) coracoid, (D) glenoid, (E) clavicle.

42. *Radiographs* (7) Normal trans-lateral.

43. *Radiographs* (8) If the patient is not able to have the arm abducted a *trans lateral* may be employed to give additional information. Detail is often poor especially in the stout patient. (A) Scapular spine, (B) glenoid, (C) coracoid, (D) A-C joints and superimposed clavicular shadows. Note the parabolic curve formed by the humeral shaft and the lateral border of the scapula.

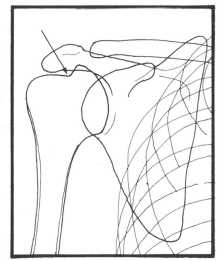

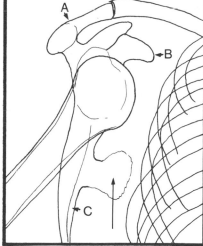

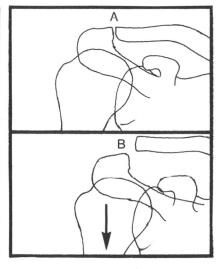

44. *Radiographs* (9) In suspected recurrent dislocation of the shoulder, an additional A-P view should always be taken with the arm internally rotated. This may show a confirmatory defect in the postero-lateral part of the head ('hatchet head'). An axial lateral will help to confirm this.

45. *Radiographs* (10) In cases of clicking or snapping shoulder, tangential views of the blade of the scapula will reveal any causal exostosis, particularly on the costal surface. (A) Acromion, (B) glenoid, (C) blade of scapula.

46. *Radiographs* (11) Where subluxation of the acromio-clavicular joint is suspected, it is *essential* that the A-P view of the shoulder is taken with the patient erect and holding a weight on the affected side. (A) Normal joint, (B) acromio-clavicular dislocation.

4 The Elbow

Tennis elbow

This is by far the commonest cause of elbow pain in patients attending orthopaedic clinics. It is generally believed to be a strain of the common extensor origin but fibrosis in extensor carpi radialis brevis or an entrapement syndrome have been suggested. The patient, usually in the 35 to 50 age group, complains of pain on the lateral side of the elbow and difficulty in holding any heavy object at arm's length. There may be a history of recent excessive activity involving the elbow — e.g. dusting, sweeping, painting or even playing tennis. Symptoms are usually relieved by 1–3 injections of local anaesthetic and hydrocortisone into the painful area. In resistant cases, local ultrasound may be tried. When all conservative measures fail, exploration of extensor carpi radialis brevis may be considered (with excision of any fibrous mass or lengthening of the tendon).

In golfer's elbow, there is a similar history, but pain and tenderness involve the common flexor origin on the medial side of the elbow. This condition is much less common than tennis elbow.

Cubitus varus and cubitus valgus

Decrease or increase in the carrying angle of the elbow generally follows a supracondylar or other elbow fracture in childhood. While the normal child has great powers of spontaneous recovery following injury, there may nevertheless be some epiphyseal damage which fails to correct; where there is evidence of interference with the carrying angle the child should be observed for a number of years. If there is failure of spontaneous correction or even deterioration, and the deformity is very unsightly, correction by osteotomy may be undertaken. In later life either of these deformities may be followed by a tardy ulnar nerve palsy.

Tardy ulnar nerve palsy

This ulnar nerve palsy is of slow onset and progression. It appears usually between the ages of 30 and 50, and the preceding injury to the elbow, considered responsible for the ischaemic and fibrotic changes in the nerve, has usually been in childhood. It is seen most frequently where there is a cubitus valgus deformity. The progress of the palsy may be arrested by transposition of the nerve from its normal position behind the medial epicondyle to the front of the joint.

Ulnar neuritis and the ulnar tunnel syndrome

Ulnar neuritis with its frequent accompaniment of small muscle wasting and sensory impairment in the hand may occur as a complication of local trauma at the elbow or at the wrist. At the elbow, it is also seen where the nerve is abnormally mobile. In these circumstances it is exposed to frictional damage as it slips repeatedly in front of and behind the medial epicondyle. In such cases re-anchorage or transposition may prevent further deterioration.

The nerve is also subject to pressure as it passes between the two heads of flexor carpi ulnaris below the elbow, or as it lies in the ulnar tunnel in the hand. Where the local findings are not clear enough to localise the site of involvement, nerve conduction rate studies are often most helpful.

In a number of cases no obvious cause for an ulnar neuritis may be found.

Olecranon bursitis

Swelling of the olecranon bursa is common in carpet-layers and others who repeatedly traumatise the posterior aspect of the elbow joint. Swelling of the bursa is also common in rheumatoid arthritis, and there may be associated nodular masses in the proximal part of the forearm. The condition is usually painless unless there is an associated bacterial infection within the bursa. Excision is sometimes advised for cosmetic reasons.

Pulled elbow

This condition occurs in young children under the age of 5, and is produced by traction on the arm, as for example when a mother snatches the hand of a child wandering towards the edge of a pavement. The radial head slides out from under cover of the orbicular ligament, and the child complains of pain and limitation of supination. The orbicular ligament and radial head may be reduced by forced supination while pushing the radius in a proximal direction; spontaneous reduction occurs usually within 48 hours of the incident if the arm is rested in a sling without manipulation.

O-A and R-A

Primary osteo-arthritis of the elbow joint is not uncommon in heavy manual labourers. O-A is also seen secondary to old fractures involving the articular surfaces; it may also follow osteochondritis dissecans. Both O-A and osteochondritis dissecans may give rise to the formation of loose bodies which restrict movements or cause locking of the joint.

R-A may affect either one or both elbows. If both elbows are involved, the functional disablement may be great.

The treatment of osteochondritis dissecans follows the same lines employed in the knee joint. Osteo-arthritic loose bodies are always removed to prevent further damage. Where there is severe functional disablement, as for example in bilateral R-A, arthroplasty may be considered.

Tuberculosis of the elbow

Tuberculosis of the elbow is now very uncommon; marked swelling of the elbow with profound local muscle wasting is usually so striking that there is unlikely to be delay in further investigation by aspiration and synovial biopsy.

Myositis ossificans

This condition occurs most commonly after supracondylar fractures and dislocations of the elbow. Calcification occurs in haematoma which forms in the brachialis muscle which covers the anterior aspect of the elbow joint. It is particularly common in association with head injuries, and may also follow over-vigorous physiotherapy. It leads to a mechanical block to flexion. If discovered at an early stage, complete rest of the joint is necessary to minimise the mass of material formed. In later cases it may be excised after the lesion has appeared quiescent for many months.

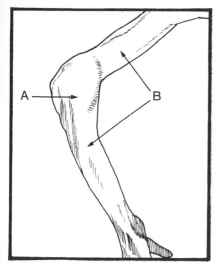

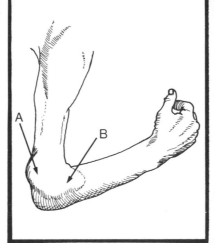

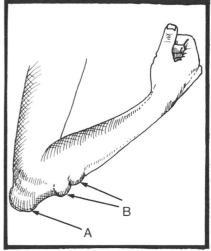

1. *Inspection:* (1) Look for (A) generalised swelling of the joint, (B) muscle wasting, both suggestive of infective arthritis (e.g. tuberculosis) or rheumatoid arthritis. The swollen elbow is always held in the semi-flexed position.

2. *Inspection:* (2) (A) Note that the earliest sign of effusion is the filling out of the hollows seen in the flexed elbow above the olecranon. (B) The next sign is swelling of the radio-humeral joint. Fluid may be squeezed between these two areas.

3. *Inspection:* (3) Note if there are any localised swellings round the joint—e.g. (A) olecranon bursitis, (B) rheumatoid nodules.

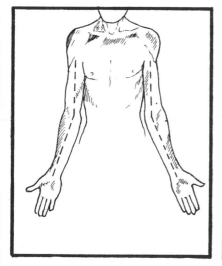

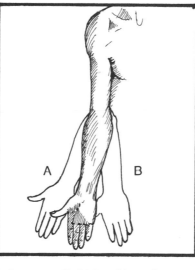

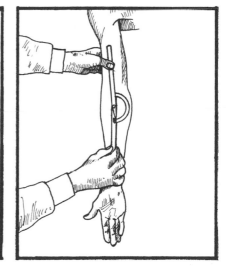

4. *Inspection:* (4) Ask the patient to extend both elbows and note the carrying angle on both sides. Any small difference between the sides will then be obvious.

5. *Inspection:* (5) (A) In cubitus valgus there is an increase in the carrying angle. (B) In cubitus varus there is a decrease in the carrying angle. The commonest cause of unilateral alteration in the carrying angle is an old supracondylar fracture.

6. *Inspection:* (6) The carrying angle may be measured with the goniometer. Average values:
Males: 11°(range 2° 26°)
Females: 13° (range 2°–22°).

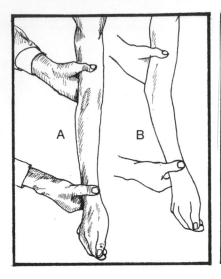

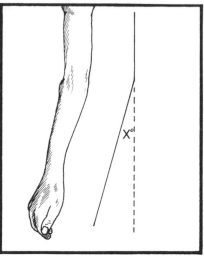

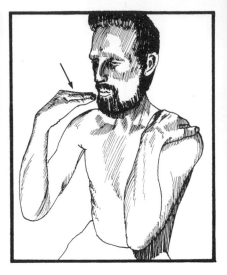

7. *Movements* (1) *Extension:* (A) Full extension, 0°, is present if the arm and forearm can be made to lie in a straight line. (B) Loss of full extension is especially common in osteo-arthritis and old fractures (particularly of the radial head) involving the elbow joint.

8. *Movements* (2) *Hyperextension:* If the elbow can be extended beyond the neutral position, record as 'X° hyperextension'. Up to 15° is accepted as normal, especially in women. Beyond this, look for hyper-mobility in other joints (e.g. Ehlers-Danlos syndrome).

9. *Movements* (3) *Flexion:* (Screening test) Ask the patient to attempt to touch both shoulders. A slight difference in flexion between the sides is then usually obvious.

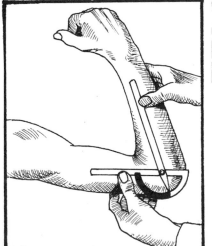

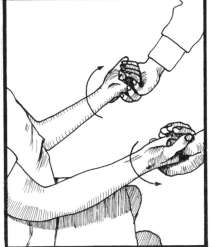

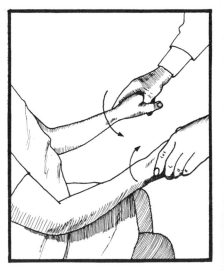

10. *Movements: Flexion* (2) The range of flexion may be measured.
Normal range = 145°
Restriction of flexion is common after all fractures round the elbow and in all forms of arthritis.

11. *Movements: Pronation/Supination Screening:* Ask the patient to hold the elbows closely to the sides. Turn the palms upwards into supination, comparing the sides.

12. *Movements: Pronation/Supination Screening* (2): Now turn the palms downwards in pronation again comparing the sides.

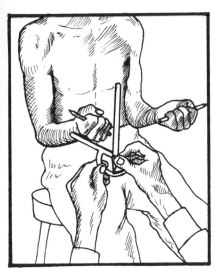

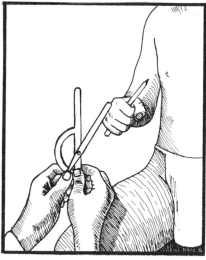

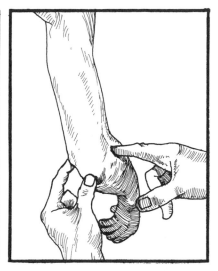

13. *Movements: Pronation:* Pronation may be recorded. Give the patient a pencil to hold, and note the angle achieved from the vertical.
Normal range = 75°

14. *Movements: Supination:* This may be measured in the same way.
Normal range = 80°
Pronation/supination movements may be reduced after fractures at the elbow, forearm and wrist (e.g. most commonly after Colles fracture). Loss may also occur after dislocation of the elbow and rheumatoid and osteo arthritis. Pure supination loss may occur in children with pulled elbow.

15. *Palpation:* (1) Begin by locating the epicondyles and the olecranon. If in doubt, flex the elbow and note the equilateral triangle normally formed by these structures. This relationship is disturbed in elbow subluxations.

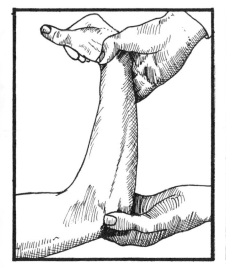

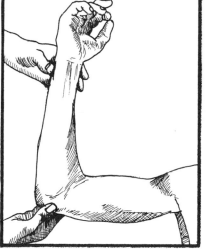

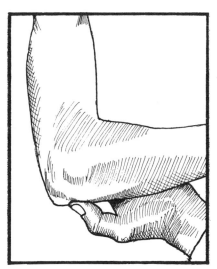

16. *Palpation:* (2) Palpate the lateral epicondyle with the thumb. Sharply localised tenderness here or just distal is almost diagnostic of tennis elbow. Carry our confirmatory tests (22). Note that after local hydrocortisone tenderness becomes more diffuse.

17. *Palpation:* (3) Palpate the medial epicondyle. Tenderness occurs here in golfer's elbow, tears of the ulnar collateral ligament, and injuries of the medial epicondyle.

18. *Palpation:* (4) Tenderness over the olecranon is uncommon, apart from fracture and infected olecranon bursitis, both of which are usually obvious.

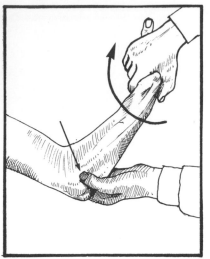

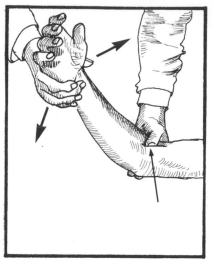

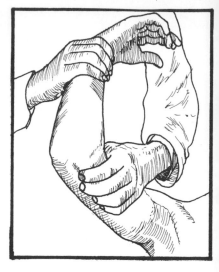

19. *Palpation:* (5) Press the thumb firmly into the space on the lateral side of the elbow between the radial head and humerus. Now pronate and supinate the arm. Tenderness here is common after injuries of the radial head, osteo-arthritis, and osteochondritis dissecans.

20. *Palpation:* (6) Palpate the front of the elbow on both sides of the biceps tendon while flexing and extending the elbow through 20°. Note the presence of any abnormal masses (e.g. myositis ossificans, loose bodies).

21. *Palpation:* (7) Roll the ulnar nerve under the fingers behind the medial epicondyle. Note if there is any difference between the sides. If indicated, carry out a fuller examination of the nerve (see *Segmental and Peripheral Nerves of the Upper Limb* 32).

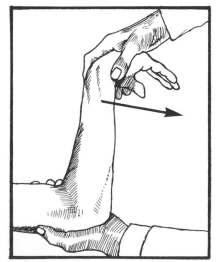

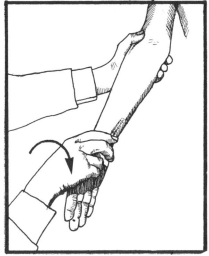

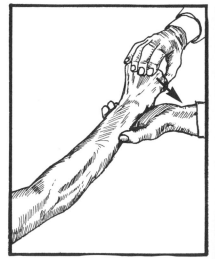

22. *Additional tests: Tennis elbow* (1) Flex the elbow and fully pronate the hand. Now extend the elbow. Pain over the lateral epicondyle is almost diagnostic of tennis elbow.

23. *Tennis elbow* (2) As an alternative, pain may be sought by pronating the arm with the elbow fully extended.

24. *Tennis elbow* (3) Ask the patient to clench the fist, dorsiflex the wrist, and extend the elbow. Try to force the hand into palmar flexion while the patient resists. Severe pain over the external epicondyle is again most suggestive of tennis elbow.

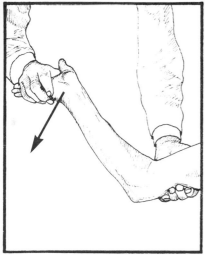

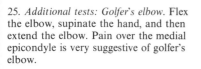

25. *Additional tests: Golfer's elbow.* Flex the elbow, supinate the hand, and then extend the elbow. Pain over the medial epicondyle is very suggestive of golfer's elbow.

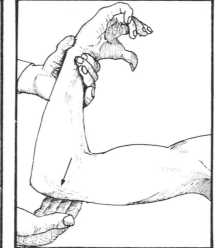

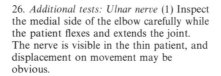

26. *Additional tests: Ulnar nerve* (1) Inspect the medial side of the elbow carefully while the patient flexes and extends the joint. The nerve is visible in the thin patient, and displacement on movement may be obvious.

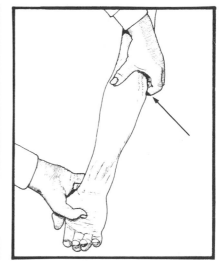

27. *Ulnar nerve* (2) Palpate again and note the extent of any tenderness, and whether the nerve is thickened. Look again for cubitus valgus. Look for evidence of ulnar nerve palsy (see *Segmental and Peripheral Nerves of Upper Limb* 32).

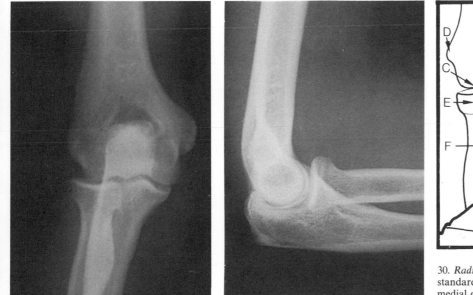

28. *Radiographs* (1) Normal A-P radiograph of the elbow.

29. *Radiographs* (2) Normal lateral radiograph of the elbow.

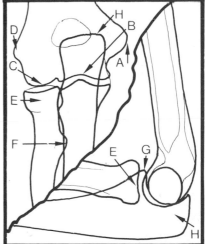

30. *Radiographs* (3) In examining the standard views, trace out the outline of (A) medial epicondyle, (B) trochlea, (C) capitulum, (D) lateral epicondyle, (E) radial head, (F) radial tuberosity, (G) coronoid process of ulna, (H) olecranon. Note the relationship between the radial head and the capitulum in both views.

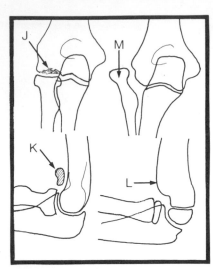

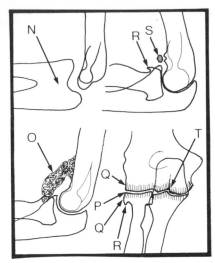

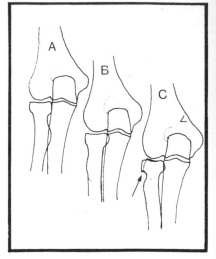

31. *Radiographs* (4) Look for (J) any defects in the capitulum suggesting osteochondritis dissecans, (K) loose bodies (usually secondary to O-A or osteochondritis), (L) incompletely remodelled supracondylar fracture (usually associated with loss of flexion), (M) Old Monteggia fracture (fracture of ulna and dislocation head of radius) usually associated with reduction of pronation and supination.

32. *Radiographs* (5) Note the presence of (N) a congenital synostosis (with inevitable loss of pronation and supination), (O) myositis ossificans (with clinically restriction of flexion). Note any osteo-arthritic changes, with for example (P) joint space narrowing, (Q) sclerosis, (R) osteophytes, (S) loose body formation, or (T) evidence of previous fracture.

33. *Radiographs* (6) Where the radial head is suspect, radiographs should be taken in the A-P plane (A) in mid-position (B) in supination (C) in pronation. These may bring an area of osteo-chondritis of the radial head or an old fracture into profile.

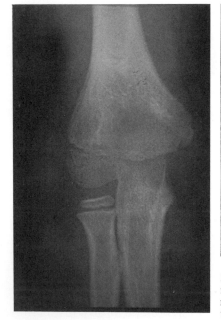

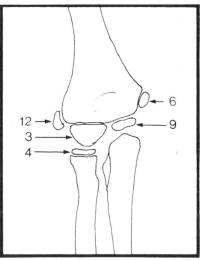

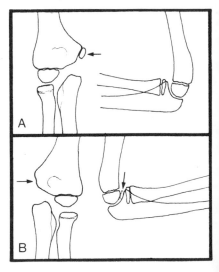

34. *Radiographs* (7) Normal A-P radiograph of the elbow of a child of 8.

35. *Radiographs* (8) Interpretation of radiographs of the elbow in children is made difficult by the changes produced by the successive appearance of ossification in the epiphyses. The old mnemonic 'cite' (capitulum, internal epicondyle, trochlea, ext. epicondyle) for appearance of the epiphyseal centres at 3, 6, 9 and 12 yrs is sufficiently accurate for normal purposes.

36. *Radiographs* (9) If there is any doubt, radiographs of both sides should be taken. Note that if a child over 6 has injured the elbow and the medial epicondyle cannot be seen, there is every likelihood it has been displaced into the joint. (A) Normal, (B) displaced.

5 The Wrist

Study of the wrist cannot be separated from the hand, and in many cases careful examination of both may be required.

Complications occurring after Colles fracture

Considering the incidence of Colles fracture, the commonest of all fractures, it is surprising that complications from this injury are not seen more frequently: nevertheless they do occur and are of importance. Excluding initial weakness of the wrist, the commonest complaints are of residual deformity, restriction of movements, and pain.

The common deformities are radial deviation of the hand and prominence of the ulna. Due to resorption of bone at the fracture site during healing, there is shortening of the radius with radial deviation of the hand. This may be aggravated by a poor reduction. At the back of the wrist, the head of the ulna becomes prominent. (Gross subluxations of the ulna of this pattern are referred to as Madelung's deformity, and this may sometimes be seen in adolescents without there being any history of trauma.)

In all Colles fractures there is disturbance of the inferior radio-ulnar joint. In some cases this is responsible for persisting pain and tenderness just lateral to the ulnar styloid.

Again, disruption of the inferior radio-ulnar joint is partly responsible for loss of movements in the wrist. This certainly accounts for the loss of supination which causes patients the greatest concern. Although restriction of dorsiflexion occurs after most Colles fractures, this seldom gives rise to any functional problems.

Two other important complications are seen after Colles fracture: (a) delayed rupture of extensor pollicis longus tendon may occur some months after injury and is due to ischaemia or attrition of the tendon and (b) Sudeck's atrophy, which is usually diagnosed some weeks after P.O.P. fixation has been discontinued, is characterised by marked swelling of the wrist, hand and fingers, gross stiffness of the fingers, and carpal decalcification which is obvious on radiographs of the region.

Regarding treatment of these complications, the patient is advised to accept minor degrees of residual deformity, and stiffness. When there is gross prominence of the ulna causing symptoms, excision of the distal end of the bone may be advised. Ruptures of extensor pollicis longus are treated by tendon transfer (extensor indicis is generally employed). Sudeck's atrophy requires intensive physiotherapy if much permanent stiffness is to be avoided.

Ganglions

Ganglions are extremely common about the wrist and hand. In many cases they may have a tenuous communication with a carpal joint or tendon sheath. Some are spherical in shape, firm, and have no obvious connection to other structures. Tiny ganglions of this type are common in the fingers. Fluctuations in the size of ganglions and their rupture from trauma is well known, and diagnosis is not usually difficult unless the swelling is small. This applies in particular to small ganglions on the back of the wrist, arising from the radio-carpal joint; local swelling and tenderness may only be obvious when the wrist is palmar flexed. This type of ganglion is often the cause of persisting wrist pain in young women: their symptoms are often labelled as functional when this difficulty in examination has not been appreciated.

Excision of most ganglions is advised.

De Quervain's disease

Tenosynovitis involving abductor pollicis longus and extensor pollicis brevis is known as De Quervain's disease. It occurs in the middle-aged. The walls of the fibrous tendon sheaths on the lateral aspect of the radius are greatly thickened, and there is often marked underlying swelling. The patient complains of pain on certain movements of the wrist, and weakness of grip. Treatment is by splitting the lateral wall of the sheath.

Extensor tenosynovitis

Acute frictional tenosynovitis occurs most frequently in the 20 to 40 age group, generally following a period of excess activity. Any or all of the extensor tendons may be involved. The condition has a benign course and usually settles if the wrist is immobilised in P.O.P. for three weeks.

O-A of the wrist

O-A of the wrist is surprisingly uncommon considering the frequency with which the joint is involved in fractures. It is seen most often after avascular necrosis of the scaphoid following fracture of that bone, non-union of the scaphoid, comminuted fractures involving the articular surface of the radius, and Kienbock's disease. (Spontaneous avascular necrosis of the lunate.)

Where symptoms are severe, fusion of the wrist (radio-carpal joint) is undertaken.

R-A

Rheumatoid arthritis of the wrist is common, and extensive synovial thickening of the joint and related tendon sheaths leads to gross swelling, increased local heat, pain and stiffness. Fluctuation can sometimes be transmitted from the wrist above the flexor retinaculum to the palm (compound palmar ganglion). Rarely tuberculosis of the wrist may produce a similar clinical picture, but the multifocal nature of rheumatoid arthritis usually makes differentiation easy.

Carpal tunnel syndrome

This condition occurs most commonly in women in the 30 to 60 age group. Basically there is compression of the median nerve which leads to symptoms and signs related to its distribution. In some cases premenstrual fluid retention, early rheumatoid arthritis with synovial tendon sheath thickening, and old carpal fractures may be responsible by restricting the space left for the nerve in the carpal tunnel. The condition is sometimes seen in association with myxoedema, acromegaly and pregnancy; often, however, no obvious cause can be found. The patient complains of paraesthesiae in the hand: often all the fingers are claimed to be involved, although theoretically at least the little finger should always be spared. Paraesthesiae may also radiate proximally to the elbow. There may be pain in the same areas, and weakness in the hand. The symptoms may become most marked in the early hours of the morning, often waking the patient from sleep and causing her to shake the hand or hang it over the side of the bed.

In many cases the history and results of the clinical examination are unequivocal. In others it may be difficult to differentiate the patient's symptoms from those produced by cervical spondylosis, and indeed both conditions may be present at the same time; a trial period of immobilisation of the wrist in P.O.P. or the use of a cervical collar may be helpful. Rarely, nerve conduction time tests may be used. Most cases are treated quite simply by division of the flexor retinaculum which forms the roof of the carpal tunnel, thereby relieving pressure on the nerve.

Ulnar tunnel syndrome

The ulnar nerve may be compressed as it passes through the ulnar carpal canal between the pisiform and the hook of the hamate. Both the sensory and motor divisions of the nerve may be affected, but often one only is involved. The symptoms therefore may include small muscle wasting and weakness in the hand with sensory disturbance on the volar aspect of the little finger. The sensory supply to the dorsum of the hand is given off in the distal forearm, so that sensory disturbance on the dorsum of the hand and little finger excludes a lesion at this level. In all cases every effort should be made to exclude a more proximal cause for the patient's symptoms (e.g. ulnar neuritis at the elbow, and cervical spondylosis.) Nerve conduction studies are often of particular value in this situation. The commonest causes of nerve involvement at the wrist are ganglionic compression, occupational trauma, ulnar artery disease and old carpal or metacarpal fractures.

On the establishment of a firm diagnosis of a localised lesion in the ulnar tunnel, exploration and decompression of the nerve are carried out.

Tuberculosis of the wrist

Tuberculosis of the wrist is now rare in Britain. Marked swelling of the joint is followed by muscle wasting in the forearm, erosion, destruction and anterior subluxation of the carpus. The diagnosis is confirmed by synovial biopsy. Monarticular rheumatism is the only condition likely to cause difficulty in diagnosis.

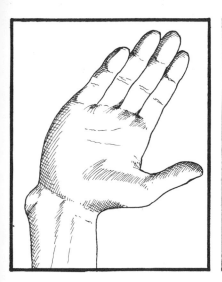

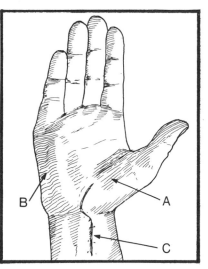

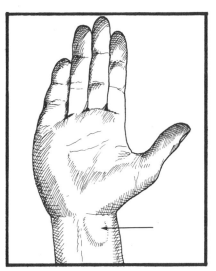

1. *Inspection: Front* (1) Note any deformity of the wrist, e.g. radial deviation of the hand, common after Colles fracture, and striking in congenital absence of the radius. Note any ulnar deviation, common in rheumatoid arthritis.

2. *Front* (2) Note (A) thenar wasting in hand, (B) hypothenar wasting, (C) scars suggestive of previous surgery or injury.

3. *Front* (3) Note any localised swellings suggestive of ganglion, rheumatoid nodule, or tumour.

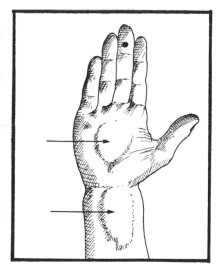

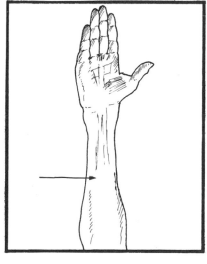

4. *Front* (4) If there is swelling at the wrist and also in the palm, try to demonstrate cross-fluctuation. This occurs in compound palmar ganglion, seen most often in rheumatoid arthritis and tuberculosis.

5. *Front* (5) Note the presence of muscle wasting in the forearm, also suggestive of R-A and tuberculosis. Widespread, bilateral wasting is common in many neurological conditions (e.g. after cervical spine injuries, multiple sclerosis etc.) and in the muscular dystrophies.

6. *Inspection Side* (1) Note any undue prominence of the ulna (common after Colles fracture or Madelung deformity) any anterior tilting of the plane of the wrist (e.g. after Smith's fracture), backward tilting (post-Colles) or anterior subluxation (TB, R-A, old carpal injury).

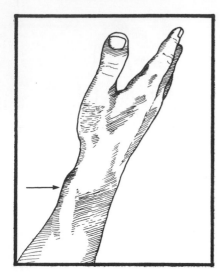

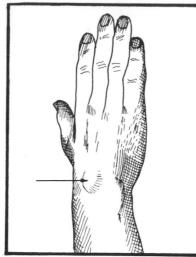

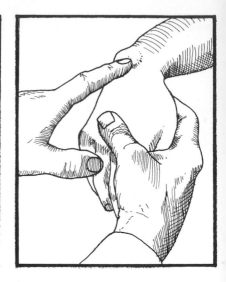

7. *Side* (1) Swelling over the lateral aspect of the distal radius occurs in De Quervain's teno-synovitis. If this is present, carry out additional tests (*Wrist* 32).

8. *Inspection: Dorsum* (1) Ganglions in relation to the wrist, carpus and extensor tendons may be quite obvious on inspection.

9. *Dorsum* (2) Palmar-flex the wrist and compare one side with the other. Small ganglions between the radius and carpus are a common source of obscure wrist pain. Palmar flexion makes such ganglions obvious, and local tenderness confirms the diagnosis.

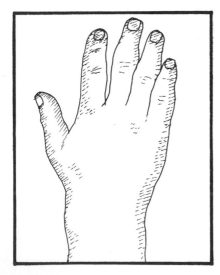

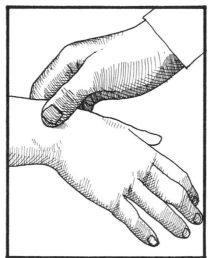

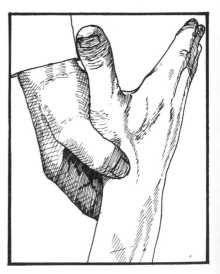

10. *Dorsum* (3) Swelling of the wrist, hand and fingers, with a glazed appearance of the skin, diffuse tenderness, pain and stiffness is typical of Sudeck's atrophy which may occur as a sequel to Colles fracture or carpal injury.

11. *Palpation* (1) Pain in the wrist persisting after a Colles fracture, and due to disruption of the inferior radio-ulnar joint is always associated with well localised tenderness at that site.

12. *Palpation* (2) Tenderness in the anatomical snuff box occurs classically after scaphoid fractures, but in fact is present after many wrist sprains and other minor injuries.

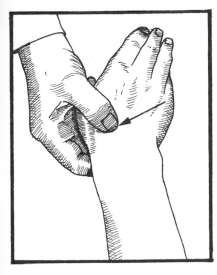

13. *Palpation* (3) To help distinguish a sprain from fracture palpate the dorsal surface of the scaphoid. Tenderness here is usually present after fractures but not sprains. Scaphoid radiographs and plaster fixation are necessary in all suspected cases of fracture.

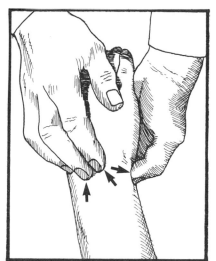

14. *Palpation* (4) Diffuse tenderness is common in all inflammatory lesions (e.g. rheumatoid arthritis and tuberculosis of the wrist) and in Sudeck's atrophy.

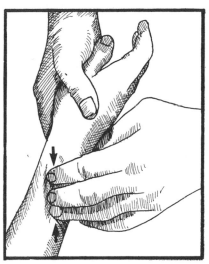

15. *Palpation* (5) Tenderness localised to the sheaths of abductor pollicis longus and extensor pollicis brevis is found in De Quervain's teno-synovitis. There is often striking local thickening of the sheaths over the dorso-lateral aspect of the radius.

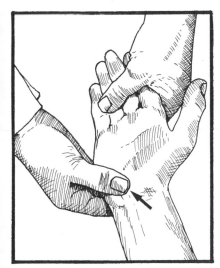

16. *Palpation* (6) Tenderness over the median nerve, with the production of paraesthesiae in the fingers and lateral side of the hand is suggestive of the carpal tunnel syndrome.

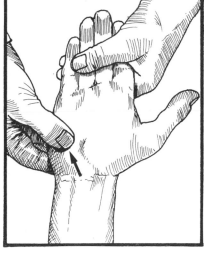

17. *Palpation* (7) In the same way, tenderness with paraesthesiae on pressure over the ulnar nerve is suggestive of the ulnar tunnel syndrome.

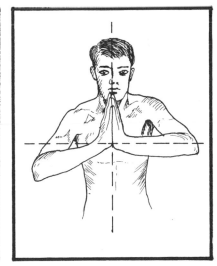

18. *Movements: Dorsiflexion* (1) *Screening test.* Ask the patient to press the hands together in the vertical plane, and to raise the elbows to the horizontal. Loss of any dorsiflexion should be obvious. The commonest cause is stiffness after a Colles fracture.

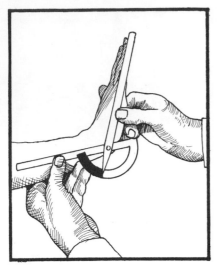

19. *Dorsiflexion* (2) Dorsiflexion may be measured with a goniometer.
Normal range = 75°
Hypermobility is not uncommon in women. If hypermobility is gross, however, other joints should be examined.

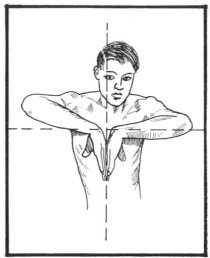

20. *Palmar Flexion* (1) *Screening Test*. Ask the patient to put the backs of the hands in contact, and then to bring the forearms into the horizontal plane. Loss of palmar flexion should be obvious.

21. *Palmar Flexion* (2) Palmar flexion may be measured with the goniometer.
Normal range = 75°

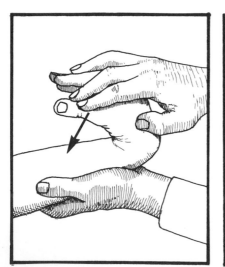

22. *Palmar Flexion* (3) If the range of palmar flexion exceeds 75°, attempt to bring the patient's thumb in line or contact with the forearm. Success indicates joint hypermobility.

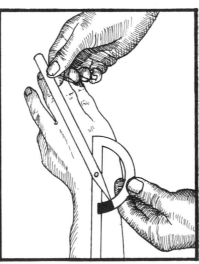

23. *Radial Deviation:* Radial deviation is measured as the angle formed between the forearm and the middle metacarpal. This test is best carried out in the mid position of the pronation/supination range.
Normal range = 20°

24. *Ulnar Deviation:* Ulnar deviation is measured in the same general way.
Normal range = 35°

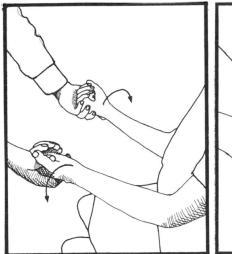

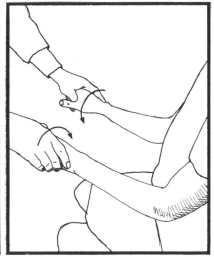

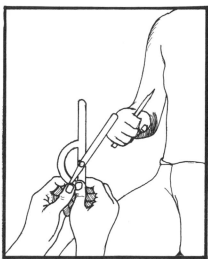

25. *Pronation/Supination: Screening test.*
Ask the patient to hold the elbows firmly at the sides. Grasp the hands and turn them so that the palms are uppernmost. Compare the amount of supination in both sides.

26. *Pronation/Supination: Screening test* (2) Repeat, turning the palms downwards to assess pronation. If no obvious cause for loss of pronation or supination is found at the wrist then the forearm and elbow must be carefully examined.

27. *Pronation:* For accurate measurement, give the patient a pen to hold. Ask the patient to keep the elbows firmly at the sides and to pronate the wrist. Measure the angle between the vertical and the held pen.
Normal range = 75°

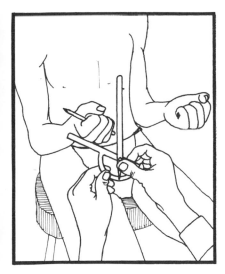

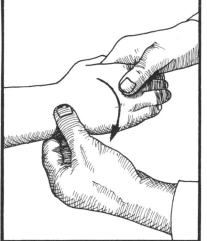

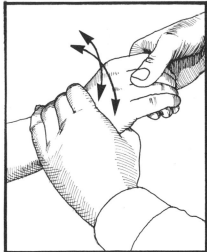

28. *Supination:* Supination may be measured in the same general way.
Normal range = 80°

29. *Crepitations: Radio-ulnar joint.* Place the index and thumb over the joint and pronate and supinate the wrist. Crepitations are common when the joint is disorganised, especially after Colles fracture.

30. *Crepitations* (2) *Radio-carpal joint.* Encircle the wrist with the hand and ask the patient to dorsiflex, palmar flex, radial deviate and ulnar deviate the wrist. Osteoarthritis of the wrist is uncommon, but occurs after scaphoid fractures, Kienbock's disease, etc.

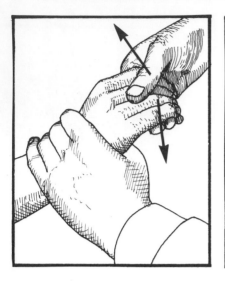

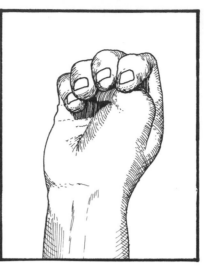

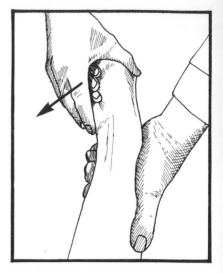

31. *Crepitations* (3) While grasping the wrist, flex and extend the fingers. Ask the patient to repeat these movements on his own. Crepitations, fine in character, occur in teno-synovitis of the extensor tendons.

32. *De Quervain's Teno-synovitis* (of abductor pollicis longus and extensor pollicis brevis). Where this is suspected from the history, local swelling and tenderness, confirm the diagnosis with the following test. Ask the patient to flex the thumb and close the fingers over it.

33. *De Quervain's Teno-synovitis* Now move the hand into ulnar deviation. Excruciating pain accompanying this manoeuvre occurs in De Quervain's teno-synovitis.

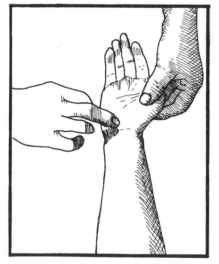

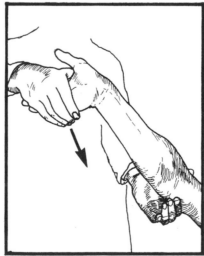

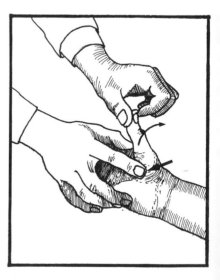

34. *Carpal Tunnel Syndrome* (1) Where this is suspected from the history, look for tenderness on pressure over the nerve (at the wrist and carpal tunnel) and for paraesthesiae on tapping the nerve.

35. *Carpal Tunnel Syndrome* (2) Note any pain and paraesthesiae on stretching the nerve by the manoeuvre of extending the elbow and dorsiflexing the wrist.

36. *Carpal Tunnel Syndrome* (3) Test the motor division of the median nerve. Note the resistance offered by patient as you try to push the vertically held thumb into the plane of the palm. Feel the thenar tone. (See also *Segmental and Peripheral Nerves of the Upper Limb* 51 *et seq.*)

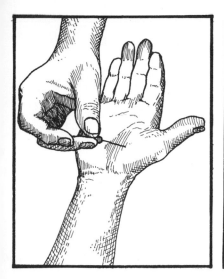

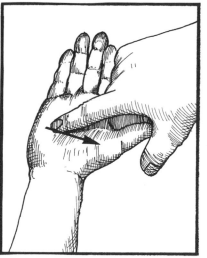

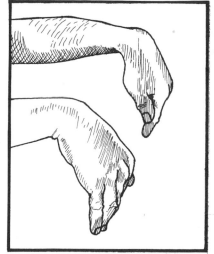

37. *Carpal Tunnel Syndrome* (4) Look for sensory impairment in the median distribution.

38. *Carpal Tunnel Syndrome* (5) Slide the tip of the index across the palm noting frictional resistance and temperature. Increased thenar resistance (from lack of sweating) and temperature rise (vaso-dilatation) may occur with median involvement.

39. *Carpal Tunnel Syndrome* (6) Ask the patient to hold both wrists in a fully flexed position for 1–2 minutes. The appearance or exacerbation of paraesthesiae is suggestive of the carpal tunnel syndrome.

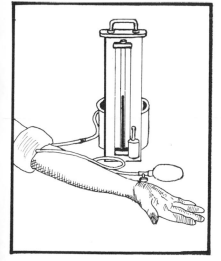

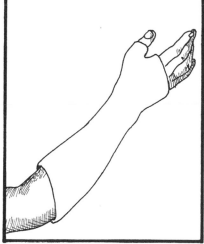

40. *Carpal Tunnel Syndrome* (7) As an alternative to the last test, apply a tourniquet and inflate to just above the systolic blood pressure for 1–2 minutes. The appearance or exacerbation of symptoms again suggests the carpal tunnel syndrome.

41. *Carpal Tunnel Syndrome* (8) If there is still doubt, apply a scaphoid plaster for 7–10 days. Improvement of symptoms while in plaster, and deterioration on removal is suggestive of the carpal tunnel syndrome.

42. *Ulnar Tunnel Syndrome* (1) Look for tenderness over the tunnel, and signs of ulnar nerve involvement (hypothenar wasting, abduction of little finger, early clawing of the ring and little fingers; see also *Segmental and Peripheral Nerves of the Upper Limb* 31 et seq.).

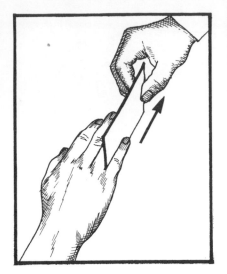

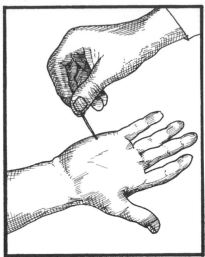

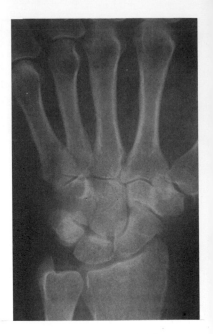

43. *Ulnar Tunnel Syndrome* (2) Test for involvement of the motor distribution of the nerve. The power of adduction of the little finger is a useful screening test.

44. *Ulnar Tunnel Syndrome* (3) Test for sensory impairment in the common area of sensory distribution of the nerve.

45. *Radiographs* (1) Normal A-P radiograph of the wrist.

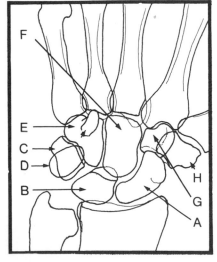

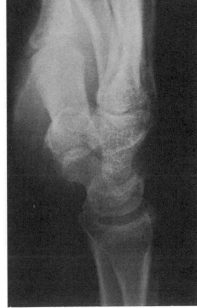

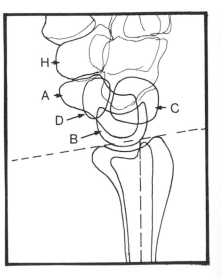

46. *Radiographs* (2) In the A-P, identify the carpal bones and note their shape, density and position. (A) scaphoid, (B) lunate, (C) triquetral, (D) pisiform, (E) hamate with hook, (F) capitate, (G) trapezoid, (H) trapezium.

47. *Radiographs* (3) Normal lateral radiograph of the wrist.

48. *Radiographs* (4) It is usually possible to make out in the lateral in spite of super-imposition, (H) trapezium, (A) tubercle and mass of scaphoid, (D) pisiform, (B) crescent of lunate, (C) triquetral. Note that the plane of the wrist joint has normally a 5° anterior tilt.

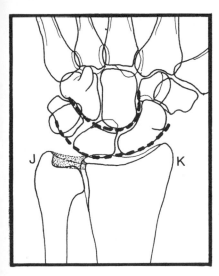

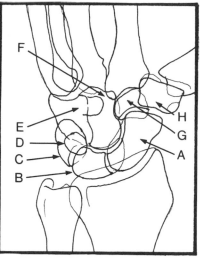

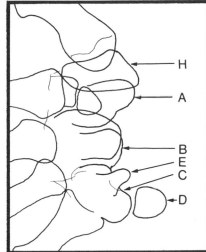

49. *Radiographs* (5) In the A-P view, note the smooth curves formed by both proximal and distal margins of scaphoid, lunate and triquetral. Note that the distal end of the ulna stops short of the radius to make room for the triangular fibro-cartilage. (J) Ulnar styloid, (K) radial styloid.

50. *Radiographs* (6) When the carpus is suspect, at least one, but preferably two oblique views should be taken in addition to the routine A-P and lateral. These are of particular value in detecting hair-line crack fractures of the carpal bones. (Key as in previous diagrams.)

51. *Radiographs* (7) In suspected carpal tunnel syndrome, a tangential projection of the tunnel should be obtained. This view occasionally shows O-A lipping or other causal pathology. (A) Scaphoid, (B) lunate, (C) triquetral, (D) pisiform, (E) hook of hamate, (H) trapezium.

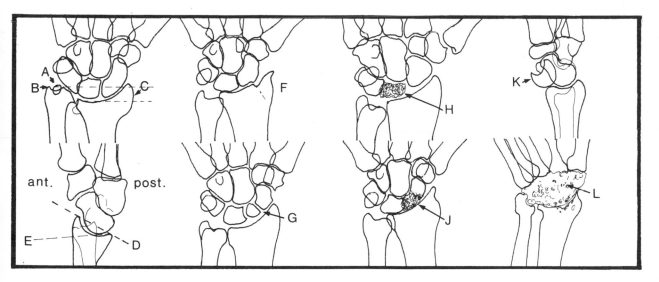

52. *Radiographs* (8) Look for evidence of previous injury. In the mal-united Colles fracture there may be (A) non-union of the ulnar styloid, (B) prominence of the distal ulna secondary to (C) distortion and resorbtion at the radial fracture. The joint line (D) may be tilted away from (E) the normal. O-A changes are uncommon after Colles fracture, but are seen in (F) radial styloid fracture. O-A may not always follow (G) non-union of a scaphoid fracture. Note increased bone density and deformity in (H) Kienbock's disease of the lunate or in (J) avascular necrosis of the scaphoid, almost invariably accompanied by O-A. Note any carpal mal-position (K), dislocation of the lunate being the most common. Gross porotic changes are seen most often in R-A and in Sudeck's atrophy, while gross destructive changes are seen in (L) TB and other infections.

6 The Hand

Note that the separation of conditions into those affecting the wrist and those affecting the hand has been done for convenience, and that in many cases examination of both regions is necessary.

Dupuytren's contracture

In this condition there is nodular thickening and contracture of the palmar fascia. The palm of the hand is affected first, and at a later stage the fingers become involved. The ring finger is most frequently affected, followed by the little and middle fingers. The index and even the thumb may be involved. In some cases there is corresponding thickening of the plantar fascia. The progressive flexion of the affected fingers interferes with the function of the hand and may be so severe that the fingernails dig into the palm. The condition affects men preponderantly over the age of 40, and in some cases there may be a hereditary tendency, or an association with epilepsy or alcoholic cirrhosis. The condition may appear in either sex at an earlier age precipitated by trauma, and then may pursue a particularly rapid course.

Surgical treatment is usually advised, but is complicated by a number of factors. If the fingers have been held in a flexed position for a long time, secondary changes in the interphalangeal joints may prevent finger extension even after the involved tissue has been removed. In the case of the fifth finger, amputation in these circumstances may be the best line of treatment. The digital nerve sheaths may blend with the fascia so that dissection is tedious and difficult; involvement of the skin may necessitate Z-plasties or other plastic procedures; and the patient's age and general health may be adverse factors. In most cases, wide excision of the affected palmar fascia is advised. When this is not possible, improvement in function, often lasting for some years, may follow simple division of the contracted fascia in the palm.

Tendon and tendon sheath lesions

See also under R-A in this section.

  a. Mallet finger. In a mallet finger the DIP joint is held in a permanent position of flexion; this may be moderate or complete. The patient is unable to extend the distal joint of the finger. The extensor tendon tears close to its attachment to the distal phalanx, or may avulse a fragment of the terminal phalanx as a result of trauma. Healing may occur spontaneously over a 6 to 12 month period, but it is usual practice to treat these injuries for six weeks with a light splint which holds the DIP joint in hyperextension.

b. Mallet thumb. Delayed rupture of the EPL tendon may follow Colles fracture (see *Wrist*) or R-A, and repair by tendon transfer (using extensor indicis proprius) is usually advised. If the tendon is damaged by an incised wound, repair by direct suture is undertaken.

c. Boutonniere deformity: Flexion of the IP joint of a finger with extension of the DIP joint characterises this deformity which is due to detachment of the central slip of the extensor tendon which is attached to the base of the middle phalanx. This may follow incised wounds on the dorsum of the finger and avulsion injuries, but is commonly seen in R-A. Surgical repair of the extensor band is often undertaken for isolated lesions of this type.

d. Extensor tendon division in the back of the hand. Extensor tendons divided by wounds on the back of the hand carry an excellent prognosis and are treated by primary suture and splintage for approximately four weeks.

e. Profundus tendon injuries

(i) Isolated avulsion injuries, which are uncommon, may be treated by surgical re-attachment of the tendon.

(ii) Profundus tendon division in open wounds: in the palm repair by direct suture is usually feasible. In the flexor tendon sheaths, there is considerable risk of adhesions spoiling function. Where finger wounds are accompanied by flexor tendon division, in many centres the skin wound only is closed and at a later date, an attempt is made to restore flexor function by employing a free flexor tendon graft. In uncontaminated wounds where good facilities are available, primary flexor tendon repair may also be undertaken. Accompanying digital nerve divisions may also be dealt with by primary repair.

f. Trigger finger and thumb. This condition results from thickening of a fibrous tendon sheath or nodular thickening in a flexor tendon.

In young children, the thumb is held flexed at the MP joint, and a nodular thickening in front of the MP joint is palpable: not infrequently the deformity is wrongly considered congenital and untreatable.

In adults, the middle or ring finger is most frequently involved. When the fingers are extended, the affected finger lags behind and then quite suddenly straightens. Nodular thickening, always at the level of the MP joint, may also be palpable. Division of the sheath at the level of the MP joint gives an immediate and gratifying cure.

Rheumatoid arthritis

Rheumatoid arthritis as is well known very frequently affects the hand, and as it progresses may involve joints, tendons, muscles, nerves and arteries, producing most severe deformities and crippling effects on hand function.

In the earliest phases the hands are strikingly warm and moist; later the joints become obviously swollen and tender. Synovial tendon sheath and joint thickening with effusion, muscle wasting, and deformity then become apparent. Tendon rupture and joint subluxation are the main factors leading to the more severe deformities.

The surgery of the rheumatoid hand is highly specialised, requiring particular skills and experience in judgement, timing and technique and is difficult to summarise with any accuracy.

In the earliest stages of the disease analgesic and anti-inflammatory drugs however are advised, with the judicious use of physiotherapy and splintage to alleviate pain, preserve movement, and minimise deformity. When there is much synovial thickening at a stage before joint destruction, synovectomy is often helpful in alleviating pain and delaying local progress of the condition. In a few well selected cases, where there is joint destruction and progressive deformity, joint replacement may be helpful; some cases of major tendon involvement may benefit from repair and other procedures.

Osteo-arthritis. IP joints

Nodular swellings (Heberden's nodes) sited over the dorsal surface of the bases of the distal phalanges (and less commonly, the middle phalanges) are a sign of osteo-arthritis of the finger joints. They occur most frequently in women after the menopause, and are often familial. They are not related to osteo-arthritis elsewhere. In most cases they are symptom-free, but may be associated with progressive joint damage and consequent pain.

Carpo-metacarpal joint of the thumb

O-A changes are common between the thumb metacarpal and trapezium and may give rise to disabling pain and impaired function in the hand. There may on occasion be a history of a previous Bennett's fracture or of occupational overuse. Several surgical procedures (e.g. excision of the trapezium) are available which give relief of pain, sometimes at the expense of some functional loss.

Tumours in the hand

Tumours in the hand are not uncommon. Most involve the soft tissues and are simple, but it need hardly be stressed that where the diagnosis is uncertain a full investigation is essential. Among the commonest tumours are the following:

1. Ganglions occur in the fingers, most commonly along the volar aspects. They are small, spherical, and tender to the touch.

2. Implantation dermoids occur along the volar surfaces of the fingers and palms.

3. Glomus tumours are less common. They are small vascular tumours, exquisitely tender and are seen most often in the region of the nail beds.

4. Enchondromata are common in the hands, may be multiple, and are often a cause of pathological fracture. Their presence may not be noted until a radiograph of the hand is taken after fracture, but in other cases there may be gross swelling and deformity.

Infections in the hand

1. Paronychia. This is the commonest of all infections in the hand, and occurs between the base of the nail and the cuticle.

2. Apical infections occur between the tip of the nail and the underlying nail bed.

3. Pulp infections occur in the fibro-fatty tissue of the finger tips, and are extremely painful. If unchecked, infection frequently leads to involvement of the terminal phalanx.

These three common infections are treated along well established lines, using antibiotics and surgical drainage if frank pus is formed.

4. Tendon sheath infections. Infection within a tendon sheath leads to rapid swelling of the finger and build up of pressure within the tendon sheath; there is always a serious risk of tendon sloughing or disabling adhesion formation. In the case of the fifth finger there may be retrograde spread of infection to involve the ulnar bursa in the hand. In the case of the thumb, infection may also spread proximally to involve the radial bursa. In either case, swelling appears in the palm and in the wrist proximal to the flexor retinaculum.

5. Web space infections. Web space infections are usually accompanied by great pain and systemic upset. There is redness and swelling in the affected web space. Infection may spread along the volar aspects of the related fingers or to adjacent web spaces across the anterior aspect of the palm. If seen early, most web space infections respond to antibiotics, splintage and elevation but drainage is sometimes necessary.

6. Mid-palmar and thenar space infections. These two compartments of the hand lie between the flexor tendons and the metacarpals. Infection may spread to them from web space or tendon sheath infections: dissemination through the hand is then rapid and potentially crippling. In either case, there is usually gross swelling of the hand and a severe systemic upset. Unless there is a rapid response to antibiotics, elevation and splintage, early drainage is essential for the preservation of function in the hand.

It should be noted that where splintage of the hand is advocated, that is if functional recovery is to be hoped for, the fingers should be held in a position of right angled flexion at the MP joints and extension in the interphalangeal joints.

7. Tuberculosis and syphilis. On rare occasions either of these two infections may produce spindle-shaped deformity of a finger. Spindling of a finger is much more common, however, in rheumatoid arthritis, gout or collateral ligament trauma.

8. Occupational infections. Superficial infections are common in certain trades and the following may be noted:

a. Pilo-nidal sinus in barbers
b. Erysipeloid in fishmongers and butchers
c. 'Butcher's wart' (tuberculous skin lesions) in butchers and pathologists
d. malignant pustule (anthrax) in hide sorters and tanners.

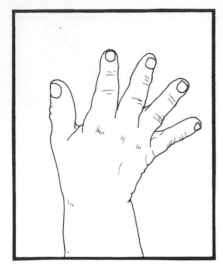

1. *Inspection.* Look first at the general shape of the hand and its size in proportion to the rest of the patient; e.g. the fingers are short and stumpy in achondroplasia. The hand is large and coarse in acromegaly. In myxoedema, the hand is often podgy and the skin dry.

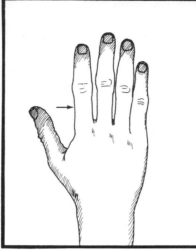

2. In Marfan's syndrome the proximal phalanges in particular are long and thin. In Turner's syndrome the ring metacarpal is often very short. In hyperparathyroidism the finger tips may be short and bulbous, while in Down's and Hurler's syndromes the little fingers are incurved.

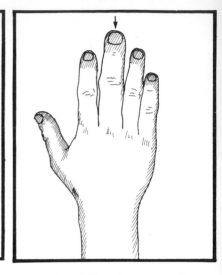

3. *Inspection* (3) Note the presence of any hypertrophy of a finger. This may occur in Paget's disease, neuro-fibromatosis and local arterio-venous fistula.

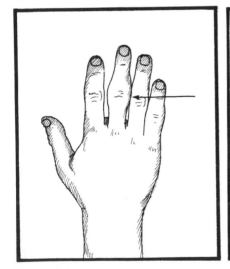

4. *Inspection* (4) Note the presence of any fusiform swelling. The commonest causes are collateral ligament tears and rheumatoid arthritis. Less commonly it is seen in syphilis, TB, sarcoidosis and gout. In psoriatic arthritis, the distal joint is usually involved.

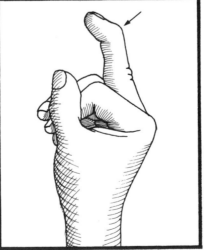

5. *Inspection: Mallet finger:* The distal inter-phalangeal joint is flexed. The patient cannot extend the terminal phalanx, although the joint can usually be extended passively. It is caused by rupture or avulsion of the extensor tendon, usually from trauma or rheumatoid arthritis.

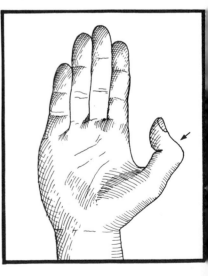

6. *Inspection: Mallet thumb:* Loss of active extension in the inter-phalangeal joint of the thumb is due to rupture of extensor pollicis longus. This is seen as a late complication of Colles fracture, from rheumatoid arthritis or wounds of the wrist or the thumb with tendon division.

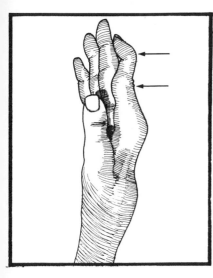

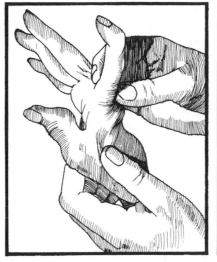

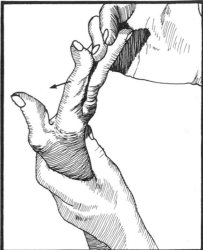

7. *Inspection: Swan-neck deformity* (1) The distal interphalangeal joint is flexed and the proximal interphalangeal joint is hyperextended. It is seen most often in rheumatoid arthritis, and may be produced by a number of different factors.

8. *Swan-neck deformity* (2) Extend the metacarpo-phalangeal joint of the affected finger. Improvement in the deformity indicates that shortening of extensor digitorum communis is a factor. If the deformity is made worse, tight interossei are likely to be responsible.

9. *Swan-neck deformity* (3) Hold all the fingers in an extended position, but leave the affected finger free. Ask the patient to flex it. If he cannot, this indicates rupture of flexor digitorum sublimis as the cause of the deformity.

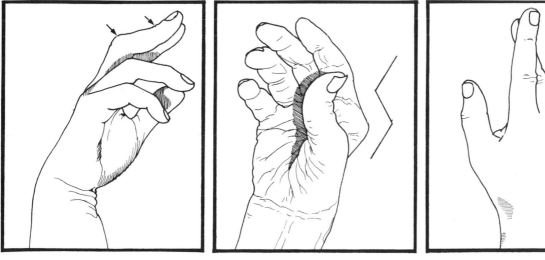

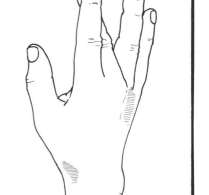

10. *Inspection: Boutonniere deformity:* The proximal interphalangeal joint is flexed and the distal joint extended. It occurs when the central extensor tendon slip to the middle phalanx is affected, by a wound on the dorsum of the finger, by traumatic avulsion, or rupture in rheumatoid arthritis.

11. *Inspection: Z-deformity of the thumb:* The thumb is flexed at the metacarpo-phalangeal joint and hyperextended at the interphalangeal joint. The deformity is seen in rheumatoid arthritis secondary to displacement of the extensor tendons or rupture of flexor pollicis longus.

12. *Inspection:* Flexion of a finger at the metacarpo-phalangeal joint, with inability to extend, follows rupture or division of the extensor tendon in the back of the hand or at the wrist.

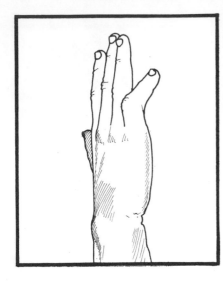

13. *Inspection:* Flexion of the little finger, mainly at the proximal inter-phalangeal joint, is seen in congenital contracture of the little finger.

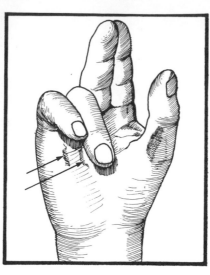

14. *Inspection:* Flexion of the fingers at the metacarpo-phalangeal and interphalangeal joints, associated with nodular thickening in the palm and fingers, is characteristic of Dupuytren's contracture. The thumb is occasionally involved.

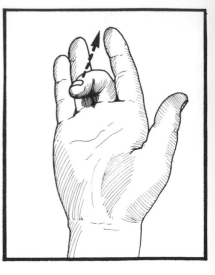

15. *Inspection:* Flexion of the middle or ring fingers at the proximal interphalangeal joint, with sudden extension on effort or with assistance, is seen in trigger finger. There is usually a palpable nodular thickening over the corresponding metacarpo-phalangeal joint.

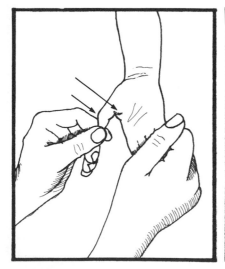

16. *Inspection:* Flexion of the interphalangeal joint of the thumb in infants and young children is usually due to stenosing teno-vaginitis involving flexor pollicis longus. A nodular thickening is usually palpable over the metacarpo-phalangeal joint.

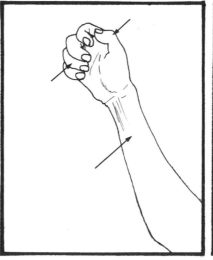

17. *Inspection:* In Volkmann's ischaemic contracture (which usually occurs as a sequel to brachial artery damage in a supracondylar fracture) there is clawing of the thumb and fingers and forearm wasting. The fingers can be extended if the wrist is flexed.

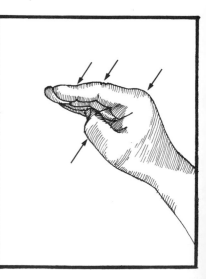

18. *Inspection:* Ischaemic contracture of the small muscles of the hand (usually as a result of swelling within a tight forearm plaster) leads to fingers which are flexed at the metacarpo-phalangeal joints and extended at the interphalangeal joints. The thumb is adducted into the palm.

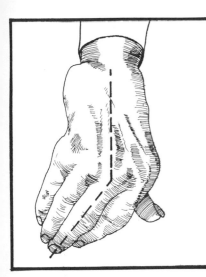

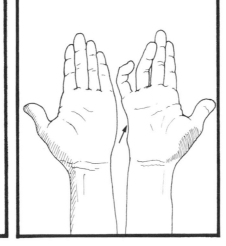

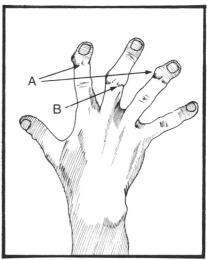

19. *Inspection:* Ulnar deviation of the fingers at the metacarpo-phalangeal joints occur in rheumatoid arthritis. In the later stages the metacarpo-phalangeal joints may dislocate.

20. *Inspection:* Unilateral wasting suggests a root, plexus or nerve lesion (see *Nerves Limb*). Widespread involvement necessitates a full examination to exlude disorders such as generalised peripheral neuropathy, syringomyelia, multiple sclerosis and the muscular dystrophies.

21. *Inspection: Swellings:* Note (A) Heberden's nodes on the dorsal surface of the distal interphalangeal joint. (They are often associated with deviation of the distal phalanx and are a sign of osteo-arthritis of the fingers.) (B) The proximal interphalangeal joints may be similarly affected (Bouchard's Nodes).

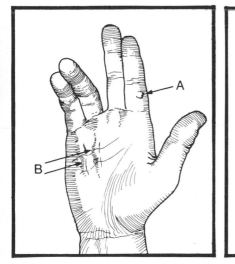

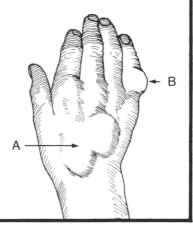

22. *Inspection: Swellings:* Note (A) firm, pea-like ganglions are common along the line of the tendon sheaths. (B) Nodular swellings of the palm and fingers accompany Dupuytren's contracture.

23. *Inspection: Swellings:* Note (A) isolated rheumatoid nodules or synovial swellings. (B) Enchondroma (sometimes multiple) is one of the commonest bone tumours occurring in the hand. If small, it may declare itself only by pathological fracture.

24. *Inspection:* Note the nutrition of the skin and nails, and the presence of finger burns or trophic ulceration, suggestive of neurological disturbance. Note any alteration of skin colour, suggesting circulatory involvement from local arterial or sympathetic supply disturbance.

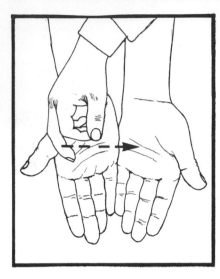

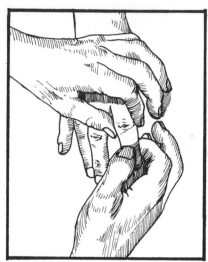

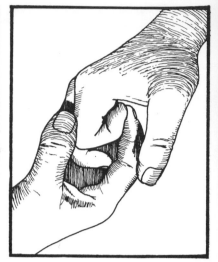

25. *Palpation* (1) Note any generalised or local disturbance of temperature or sweating in the palm or volar surfaces of the fingers. The other hand may be used for comparison.

26. *Palpation* (2) Palpate the individual finger joints between the finger and thumb, looking for thickening, tenderness, oedema and increased local heat. Note that in gouty arthritis a single joint only may be affected, especially in the early stages.

27. *Palpation* (3) Try to tuck each finger into the palm, and ask the patient to repeat unaided. Loss of active movements only is usually due to nerve or tendon discontinuity, while passive loss may be due to joint or tendon adhesions or arthritis.

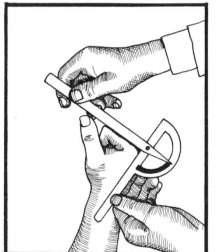

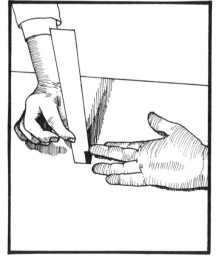

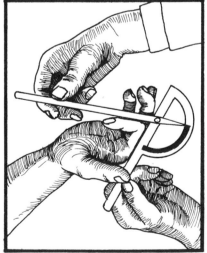

28. *Movements* (1) Where indicated for continued assessment or medico-legal purposes, both the active and passive range in an affected finger should be recorded. The normal active range in the metacarpo-phalangeal joints is 0–90°. The metacarpo-phalangeal joints can be passively hyperextended by up to 45°.

29. *Movements* (2) Extension loss may also be recorded by noting linear discrepancy. When passive extension is possible, loss of active extension suggests division, rupture or displacement of the extensor tendons, or a posterior interosseous palsy if all are affected.

30. *Movements* (3) The normal range in the proximal interphalangeal joints is 0–100°.

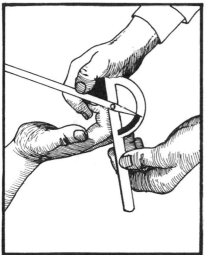

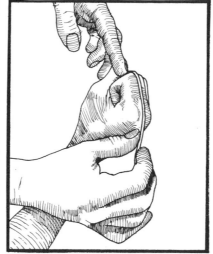

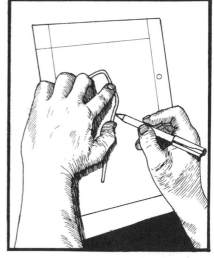

31. *Movements* (4) In the distal interphalangeal joints the normal range is 0–80°.

32. *Movements* (5) An alternative method involves moulding a length of malleable wire over the finger (14G, solder wire, approximately 2mm in diameter is suitable).

33. *Movements* (6) The wire is then transferred to the case record, and an outline drawn round it. The finger and date should be noted. An additional record of extension may be superimposed. Subsequent assessment of progress is easily made by repeating the process.

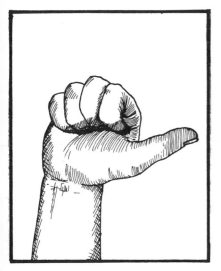

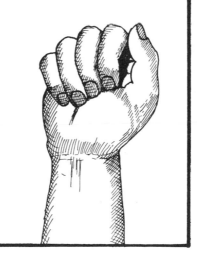

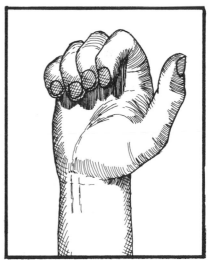

34. *Movements* (7) *Composite movement:* As all the joints of all the fingers are involved in grasping and holding, ask the patient to make a fist. Normally the distal phalanges should 'tuck-in', touching the palm at right angles.

35. *Movements* (8) Only a slight loss at any level is sufficient to prevent 'tuck-in'. All the fingers may be involved as shown. If a single finger is affected its prominence will be obvious. This screening test may be carried out earlier in the examination if desired.

36. *Movements* (9) Greater reduction in movements will prevent the fingers from reaching the palm, and indicate more serious impairment of the patient's ability to grasp and hold.

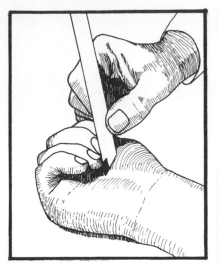

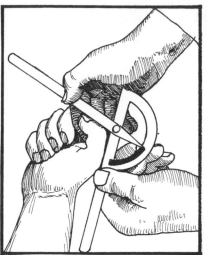

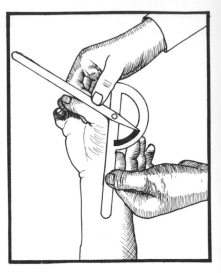

37. *Movements* (10) This important restriction of functional ability may be measured by noting the distance that the fingers stand proud of the palm on maximum flexion.

38. *Movements* (11) *The thumb:* The normal inter-phalangeal joint can be flexed 80° and extended 20° (both actively and passively) beyond the neutral position, giving a total range of 100°.

39. *Movements* (12) The normal range of flexion in the metacarpo-phalangeal joint is approximately 55°. The joint may be extended passively 5° beyond the neutral position.

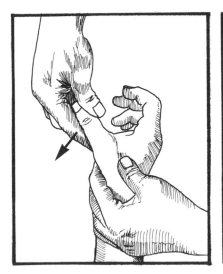

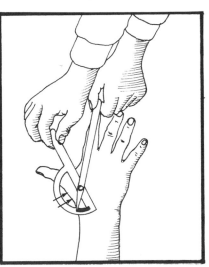

40. *Movements* (13) At this stage, test the stability of the metacarpo-phalangeal joint in a side-to-side plane. Extend the joint and stress the medial collateral ligament. Compare the sides. Excess mobility follows tears ('gamekeeper's thumb') and rheumatoid arthritis and can be very disabling.

41. *Movements* (14) *Carpo-metacarpal joint:* Test extension (abduction parallel to the plane of the palm) by placing the hand palm down, and measuring the range from a position in contact with the index to its fully extended position.
Normal range = 20°

42. *Movements* (15) *Carpo-metacarpal flexion:* From the neutral position with the thumb in contact with the index, the normal thumb can flex 15°. This angle is difficult to measure, and an accurate assessment is seldom of value.

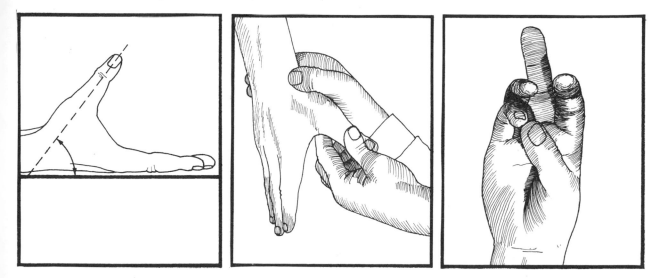

43. *Movements* (16) *Abduction of the thumb in a plane at right angles to the palm:* The patient attempts to point the thumb at the ceiling, with the back of the hand resting on a table.
Normal range = 60°

44. *Movements* (17) While examining the carpo-metacarpal joint of the thumb, note any crepitations from the joint. This finding is common in osteo-arthritis and rheumatoid arthritis of this joint, and there is often prominence of the base of the metacarpal.

45. *Movements* (18) *Opposition* (1) This movement involves abduction at right angles to the palm, flexion, and rotation. Normally the thumb should be able to touch the tip of the little finger.

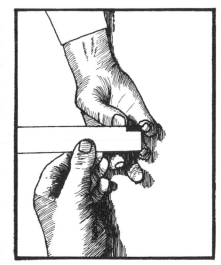

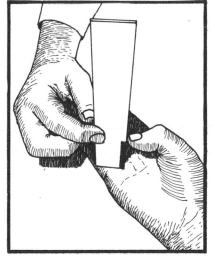

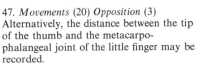

46. *Movements* (19) *Opposition* (2) Loss of opposition may be assessed by measuring the distance between the tip of the thumb and little finger.

47. *Movements* (20) *Opposition* (3) Alternatively, the distance between the tip of the thumb and the metacarpo-phalangeal joint of the little finger may be recorded.

48. *Movements* (21) Finger abduction may be assessed by measuring the spread between index and little fingers, or the spread between individual fingers.

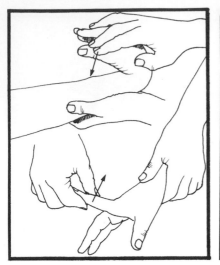

49. *Movements* (22) *Hypermobility:* Try to bring the thumb against the radius, or note hyperextension at the metacarpo-phalangeal joints of the fingers. Hypermobility occurs in the Ehlers-Danlos syndrome, Marfan's syndrome, osteogenesis imperfecta and Morquio-Brailsford's disease.

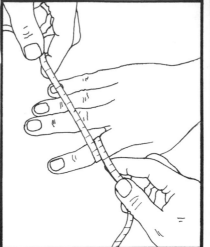

50. *Joint thickening and swelling.* The activity of the inflammatory process in a swollen joint is sometimes assessed by measuring the joint circumference from time to time. Accuracy without special equipment is difficult to achieve, and the results of limited value.

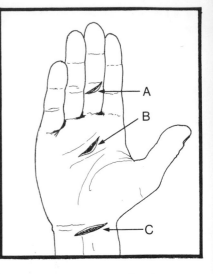

51. *Tendon injuries* (1) Note first the position of any wound, and try to work out the structures at risk, e.g. (A) flexor profundus, (B) sublimis, and if deeper, profundus, (C) median nerve, flexor carpi radialis longus, sublimis, and more deeply profundus tendons.

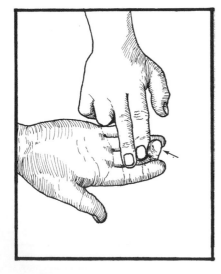

52. *Tendon injuries* (2) If the *profundus* tendon is suspect, support the finger and ask the patient to bend the tip. Loss of the ability to flex the terminal phalanx occurs when the flexor digitorum profundus tendon is divided.

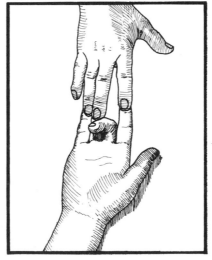

53. *Tendon injuries* (3) If the *sublimis* tendon is suspect, hold all the fingers except the suspect one in a fully extended position to neutralise the effect of flexor profundus. If the patient is able to flex the finger at the proximal interphalangeal joint then sublimis is intact.

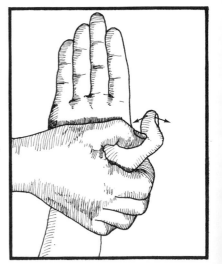

54. *Tendon injuries* (4) *Flexor and extensor pollicis longus:* Support the proximal phalanx and ask the patient to flex and extend the tip.

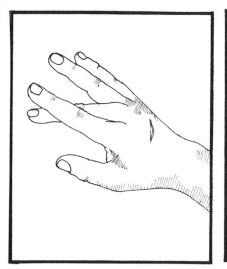

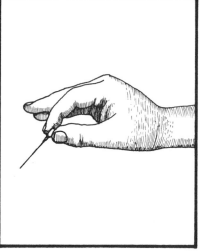

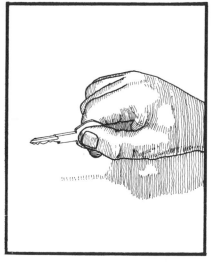

55. *Tendon injuries (5) Extensor digitorum communis:* Ask the patient to extend the fingers. Any extensor tendon divided on the dorsum of the hand or finger will be obvious by the lack of extension in the finger, assuming the finger joints have been checked for mobility.

56. *Assessment of the principal functions of the hand: Pinch grip:* Ask the patient to pick up a small object between the tips of the thumb and index. Intact sensation is necessary for a satisfactory performance. The patient should be asked to repeat the test with his eyes closed.

57. *Hand function (2) Thumb to side of index grip:* The patient should be asked to grip a key between the thumb and side of the index in the normal fashion. Test the firmness of the grip by attempting to withdraw the key, using your own pinch grip.

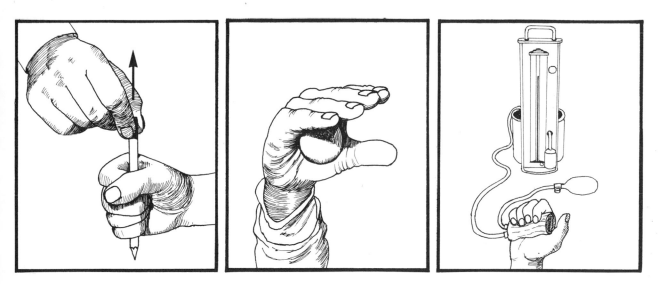

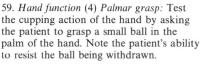

58. *Hand function (3) Grasp:* Ask the patient to grasp a pen firmly in the hand, using the thumb and fingers. Attempt to withdraw the pen and note the resistance offered. Where finger flexion is restricted, repeat using an object of greater diameter.

59. *Hand function (4) Palmar grasp:* Test the cupping action of the hand by asking the patient to grasp a small ball in the palm of the hand. Note the patient's ability to resist the ball being withdrawn.

60. *Hand function (5) Grip strength:* Inflate a rolled sphygmomanometer cuff to 20 mm of mercury and ask the patient to squeeze it as hard as he can. A reading of 200 mm or over should be achievable with the normal hand.

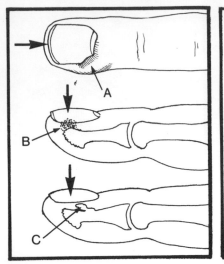

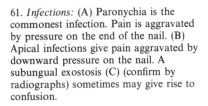

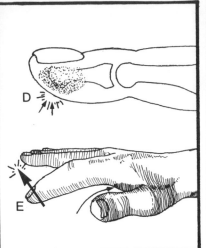

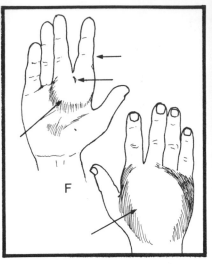

61. *Infections:* (A) Paronychia is the commonest infection. Pain is aggravated by pressure on the end of the nail. (B) Apical infections give pain aggravated by downward pressure on the nail. A subungual exostosis (C) (confirm by radiographs) sometimes may give rise to confusion.

62. *Infections:* (D) Pulp infections are exquisitely tender and may lead to destruction of the distal phalanx. (E) Tendon sheath infections lead to a fusiform flexed finger. Straightening causes pain. Tenderness is marked and localised (usually to the base of the sheath).

63. *Infections:* (F) In web space infections, there is usually marked swelling of the back of the hand and web, with spreading of the fingers. Note the site of any causal wound.

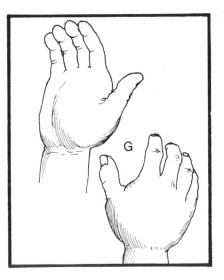

64. *Infections:* (G) In thenar and mid-palmar space infections there is gross swelling of the hand involving both the dorsal and palmar surfaces. In the case of the thenar space, the swelling may be more pronounced on the radial side of the palm.

7 The Thoracic and Lumbar Spine

Low back pain is by far the commonest spinal complaint. In the majority of cases this is due to a prolapsed lumbar intervertebral disc, osteo-arthritis of the spine, or 'low back strain'. The rarer conditions affecting the spine may give rise primarily or secondarily to lumbar backache; these less common conditions must be eliminated in every case, as there are so many essential differences in their prognosis and management.

Scoliosis

Scoliosis is a lateral curvature of the spine. In the management of any case, the first and most important decision to make is whether there is any deformity of the vertebrae (structural scoliosis). If the vertebrae are normal (non-structural scoliosis) the deformity is usually due to one of the following conditions: it may be *compensatory*, resulting from tilting of the pelvis from real or apparent shortening of one leg. It may be *sciatic*, and due to unilateral protective muscle spasm especially accompanying a prolapsed intervertebral disc. *Postural* scoliosis occurs most commonly in adolescent girls and generally resolves spontaneously.

In *structural scoliosis* there is alteration in vetebral shape and mobility, and the deformity cannot be corrected by alteration of posture. A careful history and examination is required to find a cause and give a prognosis, the two factors on which treatment depends. Structural scoliosis may be *congenital*, the deformity being due for example to a hemivertebra (only half of a single vertebra is fully formed), fused vertebrae or absent or fused ribs.

In *paralytic* scoliosis the deformity is secondary to loss of the supportive action of the trunk and spinal muscles, nearly always as a sequel to anterior poliomyelitis.

Neuropathic scoliosis is seen as a complication of neurofibromatosis, cerebral palsy, spina bifida, syringomyelia, Freidrich's ataxia and neuropathic conditions. Primary disorders of the supportive musculature of the spine are responsible for *myopathic scoliosis* (e.g. in muscular dystrophy, arthrogryphosis). *Metabolic scoliosis* is uncommon, but occurs in Cystine storage disease, Marfan's syndrome and rickets. *Idiopathic scoliosis* is the commonest and by far the most important of the structural scolioses, and its cause remains obscure. Several vertebrae at one or less commonly two distinct levels are affected (primary curve).

71

In the area of the primary curve there is loss of mobility (the fixed curve) and *rotational* deformity of the vertebrae (the spinous processes rotate into the concavity, and the bodies which carry the ribs in the thoracic region rotate into the convexity). Above and below the fixed primary curves, *secondary curves* which are mobile develop in an effort to maintain the normal position of the head and pelvis. The spinal deformity is accompanied by shortening of the trunk, and there is often impairment of respiratory and cardiac function. In severe cases this may lead to invalidism and shortening of life expectancy.

Once scoliosis has appeared in the growing child the natural tendency is to deterioration. The prognosis of a given case is dependent on the age of onset (deterioration after cessation of growth is uncommon, but can occur from disc degeneration and vertebral subluxation), the level of the spine affected, the size and number of the primary curves, and the type of structural scoliosis (e.g. idiopathic or congenital). Generally speaking, the higher the level of the spine involved in the primary curve, and the younger the patient, the worse the prognosis. There is the notable exception that in some cases occurring in infancy there is spontaneous recovery which is as remarkable as its mysterious onset. Favourable factors are left sided curves occurring in the first year of life in males where there is a rib-vertebral angle of less than 20°.

In all cases of structural scoliosis radiographic measurement of the curves and careful observation is essential. Treatment may be advised in the face of a poor prognosis or on evidence of rapid deterioration. The methods available are highly specialised as is the decision regarding their use and timing. Deterioration in a curve may be controlled by use of the *Milwaukee brace* (a device incorporating moulded supports for the chin, occiput and pelvis, interconnected by vertical metal struts). This support is employed in older children approaching skeletal maturity who have just acceptable curves or it may be used in the young child until an age suitable for spinal fusion (10 or over) is reached. *Fusion* of the entire primary curve is aimed at preventing further deterioration and in allowing braces to be discarded. Prior to fusion it is necessary to correct the primary deformity as much as is possible. Often a hinged plaster spica (Risser jacket) or the surgical insertion of internal apparatus (e.g. Harrington instrumentation) are employed.

Kyphosis

Kyphosis is the term used to describe an increased forward curvature of the thoracic spine, obvious when the patient is viewed from the side. (Diminution of the lumbar concave curve is referred to as loss of lumbar lordosis or flattening of the lumbar curvature; in extreme cases there is reversed lordosis, or posterior convexity of the lumbar curve.) Kyphosis generally affects the major part of the thoracic spine, and the increased curvature is usually regular. In angular kyphosis, which must be carefully distinguished, there is an abrupt alteration in the thoracic curvature which is usually accompanied by undue prominence of a spinous process (gibbus). Where mobility is normal in the kyphotic spine, the deformity is most frequently postural, occurring as in postural scoliosis most frequently in adolescent girls. In some cases the deformity is secondary to an increased lumbar lordosis (which in turn may be due to abnormal forward tilting of the pelvis, sometimes from flexion contracture of the hips or congenital dislocation of the hips). Less commonly, kyphosis may result from muscle weakness secondary to anterior poliomyelitis or muscular dystrophy.

When the thoracic curvature is not mobile but fixed, the most frequent causes are Scheuermann's disease, ankylosing spondylitis, senile kyphosis, and Paget's disease. When there is an angular kyphosis, the most common causes are tuberculous or other infections of the spine, fracture (traumatic or pathological) and in children, eosinophilic granuloma.

Scheuermann's disease (spinal osteochondrosis)

This condition, whose exact aetiology is not known, results in a growth disturbance of the thoracic vertebral bodies which in lateral radiographs of the spine are seen to be narrower anteriorly than posteriorly (anterior wedging). The body epiphyses are often irregular and may be disturbed by herniation of the nucleus pulposus. Nuclear herniation may occur between the epiphyses and bodies anteriorly, or into the centre of the bodies (Schmorl's nodes). Mobility is impaired, thoracic kyphosis is regular and often quite marked, and there is a compensatory increase in lumbar lordosis. Secondary O-A changes may supervene in the thoracic and lumbar spine. Active treatment (e.g. using Harrington instrumentation and posterior spinal fusion) is seldom advocated. The patient complains of mild thoracic backache, rounding of the shoulders, and in later life low back pain from secondary osteo-arthritis.

Calvé's disease

Back pain in children may be accompanied by gross flattening of a single vertebral body. Symptoms resolve spontaneously. In many cases the pathology seems due to an eosinophilic granuloma.

Ankylosing spondylitis

In this disease there is progressive ossification of the joints of the spine; its aetiology is unknown. The incidence is greatest in males during the third and fourth decades. Unlike R-A to which it is often related, it is comparatively rare in women. The joints between D12 and L1 are often first affected, but the rest of the thoracic and lumbar spine is rapidly involved with striking loss of mobility. The costo-vertebral joints are usually affected leading to a reduction in chest expansion and vital capacity; pulmonary tuberculosis is sometimes found as a complication. Stiffness of the back and pain are the presenting symptoms in the majority of cases, but on occasion involvement of the knees or hips may first attract attention. The disease is progressive and although it sometimes arrests spontaneously at an early stage it usually leads to complete ankylosis of the spine, with characteristic changes in the radiographs (bambooing of the spine). The sacro-iliac joints are almost invariably involved at an early stage, and there may be fusion of the manubrio-sternal joint. The sedimentation rate is high (40 to 120 mm) and there is often associated anaemia, muscle wasting and weight loss. The progress of ankylosing spondylitis may be controlled by anti-inflammatory drugs or by carefully controlled deep X-ray therapy. Where deformity of the spine is gross, spinal osteotomy is occasionally undertaken to give the patient a tolerably erect posture. Replacement arthroplasty of the hips is often undertaken if these joints have progressed to fusion.

Senile kyphosis

In true senile kyphosis, the ageing patient becomes progressively stooped and shorter in stature through degenerative thinning of the intervertebral discs. Pain may occur if there is associated osteo-arthritis.

In elderly women, the kyphosis may be aggravated by senile osteoporosis or osteomalacia which lead to anterior vertebral wedging and often pathological fracture. There is usually radiographic evidence of decalcification, the serum chemistry may be disturbed, and pain is a feature if fracture is present. Treatment is directed towards controlling the underlying osteoporosis or osteomalacia. Thoracic spinal supports are not particularly effective and cannot be tolerated by the elderly, but often a simple lumbar corset support is helpful in relieving pain arising from the associated lumbar lordosis.

Paget's disease

Paget's disease of the spine is comparatively uncommon and although the diagnosis is made on the radiographic findings, it may be suggested clinically by other stigmata of the disease.

Tuberculosis of the spine

Bone and joint tuberculosis is now uncommon in Britain, so that although the spine is involved in 50 per cent of cases, tuberculosis of the spine is now seldom seen. Nevertheless, it must never be forgotten. The onset is often slow with aching pain in the back and stiffness of the spine. Radiographs taken in the earliest stages of the disease show narrowing of a single disc space; later, as the anterior portions of the vertebral bodies become progressively involved, they collapse leading to anterior and sometimes lateral wedging of the spine. This may produce angular kyphotic or scoliotic deformities. The local abscess may expand and track distally; the spinal cord may be involved as a result of pressure from abscess and necrotic bone fragments, from spinal artery thrombosis and from spinal angulation; paraplegia may result.

Initial investigation should include radiographs of the chest, a Mantoux test, and in the case of the lumbar spine at least, an IVP (renal spread being not uncommon). The clinical and radiological features of tuberculosis of the spine are mimicked in the early stages by other infections (especially those due to the *Staphylococcus aureus*) and the only certain method of establishing the diagnosis in the majority of cases seen at this stage is by obtaining specimens for histological and bacteriological examination. As the abscess is small at first and the early removal of necrotic bone and pus is generally of value from the point of view of accelerating healing, many surgeons combine these procedures. In the later stages where there is gross bone destruction, minimal new bone formation, and the formation of large abscesses, the diagnosis is seldom in doubt. The mainstay of treatment is the prolonged use (six months to two years) of the antituberculous drugs.

A number of regimes using combinations of Streptomycin, PAS, INAH, Rifampicin, etc. are advocated, and sensitivity testing is advisable. The aim of treatment is to overcome the infection, eliminate abscesses and sequestra, and promote sound fusion in the affected spinal segment to prevent recrudescence. Where abscesses are substantial they should be evacuated surgically. Fusion may occur spontaneously, but there is at present a trend to early surgical intervention to achieve or accelerate this process. Where paraplegia complicates the disease, decompression of the cord in the early stages is often followed by partial or complete cure. In paraplegia of late onset, where the cord is often acutely angled over an internal gibbus, surgical intervention should always be carried out, but the prognosis here is less good.

Pyogenic osteitis of the spine

Pyogenic osteitis of the spine is relatively uncommon. In the early stages of the disease differentiation from tuberculosis of the spine is often extremely difficult, so that the diagnosis may not be clearly established unless material is provided for bacteriological examination. Specimens may be obtained by needle biopsy with the use of an image intensifier, or by exploration. At a later stage (and many cases may delay in their presentation) exuberant new bone formation in the region of the lesion may favour this diagnosis. The presenting features are of pain and stiffness in the back, often of insidious onset, but sometimes occurring quite rapidly. Nearly all cases resolve with prolonged treatment with the appropriate antibiotic (the majority are due to a staphylococcal infection, but *Salmonella, B. Typhosus* and other organisms are sometimes causal).

Metastatic lesions of the spine

Metastatic disease of the spine is seen particularly in the elderly and may be complicated by paraplegia. The diagnosis is radiographic. Treatment of the uncomplicated lesion is dependent on the nature of the primary tumour; in some cases deep X-ray therapy and supportive measures may help the local lesion and give relief of pain. Where paraplegia is present, decompression should be undertaken unless the case is terminal. Primary tumours of the spine are rare; the common types are mentioned in the Cervical Spine section.

Spondylolysis, spondylolisthesis

In the erect position, there is a tendency for the body of the fifth lumbar vertebra, (carrying the weight of the trunk), to slide forwards on the corresponding surface of the sacrum, as the plane of the L5–S1 disc is not horizontal but slopes downwards anteriorly. This movement is usually prevented by the downward projecting inferior articular processes of the fifth lumbar vertebra impinging on the corresponding upward projecting articular processes of the sacrum. This mechanism may fail if there is a fracture or congenital defect in the part of the fifth lumbar vertebra lying immediately anterior to its inferior articular process. A defect in this region, if unaccompanied by any significant forward movement of the vertebral body, is known as spondylolysis. The defect may be unilateral or bilateral. When forward slip occurs, the condition is known as spondylolisthesis. Less commonly, the fourth lumbar vertebra may be involved, the slip occurring between L4 and L5.

Both these conditions give rise to low back pain which radiates into the buttocks. In mild cases, symptoms may be controlled by a corset support. In more severe cases, a local spinal fusion is the treatment of choice. A number of patients may suffer from neurological disturbances in the lower limbs. These may be due to an associated disc protrustion, or be caused by the cauda equina and roots of the lumbosacral plexus being stretched over the prominent upper edge of the fifth lumbar vertebra or the sacrum. These complications are dealt with by disc excision or trimming of the prominence at the same time as local fusion.

Osteo-arthrosis (osteo-arthritis)

Primary O-A of the spine is extremely common, especially in the elderly, and is often asymptomatic. In the majority of cases there are no obvious causes, apart from those associated with the degenerative processes of age. Sometimes overweight and excessive use of the spine in manual workers may be factors. In secondary O-A, previous pathology in the spine accelerates normal wear and tear processes.

Occasionally osteo-arthritis may be localised to one spinal level at for example the site of a previous fracture or a prolapsed intervertebral disc. Often, however, many vertebral levels are affected, particularly where there is some alteration in the normal curves of the spine; for example secondary O-A changes may occur in the lumbar spine when lumbar lordosis is increased as a sequel to Scheuermann's disease of the thoracic spine.

O-A of the spine may be accompanied by disc degeneration, anterior and posterior lipping of the vertebral bodies, narrowing and lipping of the facet joints, and sometimes abuttment of the vertebral spines (kissing spines) due to approximation of the vertebrae from disc degeneration.

The symptoms of O-A are of pain and stiffness in the back, and once other conditions have been eliminated, the radiographic appearances are diagnostic.

Treatment is by weight reduction where applicable, spinal exercises to improve the back musculature, and analgesics. Short-wave diathermy is sometimes helpful. In the commonest area, the lumbar spine, a corset support is a widely used and generally very helpful line of treatment. Only rarely is spinal fusion indicated, but this is sometimes considered in the younger patient suffering from secondary osteo-arthritis involving one level only.

Rheumatoid arthritis

R-A may affect the spine: other peripheral sites are normally involved, so that the diagnosis is not normally difficult. Radiographs of the spine in R-A generally show widespread osteoporosis, disc space narrowing and narrowing of the facet joints. The treatment is that of generalised R-A; locally, corset supports may give considerable relief of symptoms.

Spina bifida

Spina bifida is a condition in which there is a congenital failure of fusion of the posterior elements of the spine, through which the contents of the spinal canal may herniate. The grosser forms in the newly born child present no difficulty in diagnosis. A number require and are amenable to immediate surgery, which may prevent early death from ascending meningitis and ameliorate the frequently concomitant neurological and hydrocephalic problems. The residual neurological defect may unfortunately be profound and the selection of cases for surgery is specialised and to some extent controversial.

The older child or adult may present with spina bifida occulta, which is diagnosed by radiological examination, although it may be suspected by the presence of a hairy patch, naevus, fat pad or dimpling of the skin at the site of the abnormality. Many cases are symptom-free. In some the only manifestation may be the presence of pes cavus. In others there may be progressive bladder dysfunction, weakness and inco-ordination of the legs, or trophic changes in the feet.

Spinal stenosis

A decrease in the sagittal diameter of the spinal canal, perhaps associated with narrowing of the nerve root tunnels may give rise to symptoms of vague backache and morning stiffness. Occasionally there may be temporary motor paralysis or neurogenic claudication where there are lower limb pains, cramps and paraesthesiae related to walking or exercise. There may be weakness or giving-way of the legs. The claudication distance is variable and the sensory loss segmental;

impulse symptoms are usually present. (In claudication due to vascular insufficiency, the claudication distance is constant, the peripheral pulses are usually absent, and the sensory loss generally of stocking type.)

Spinal stenosis is common in achondroplasia. In others the condition may be suspected on clinical grounds; the diagnosis may often be confirmed by computer assisted tomography, although analysis of the dimensions of the pedicles and the spinal canal and myelography may be helpful.

The prolapsed intervertebral disc

Disc prolapse is rare in the thoracic region, and at this level diagnosis is difficult without myelography. Lumbar disc prolapses on the other hand are common, and the diagnosis is usually made on the clinical evidence alone. Confirmation is not normally made by myelography unless exploration is being considered or if any of the features of the case raise the possibility of an intrathecal tumour or other pathology.

The disc between L5 and S1 is most commonly involved followed in order by L4–L5, and that between L3 and L4. In a typical case there is a history of a flexion injury which tears the annulus fibrosus, allowing the nucleus pulposus to herniate through. Back pain is produced by the annular tear and protective lumbar muscle spasm may contribute to it. Pain is felt in the lumbar region. There is usually tenderness between the spines at the affected level, and sometimes at the side over muscles in spasm. Muscle spasm often leads to loss of the normal lumbar lordotic curve, to restriction of movements in the lumbar spine, and a protective scoliosis. The extruding nucleus frequently presses on a lumbar nerve root, giving rise to sciatic pain, paraesthesiae in the leg, and sometimes muscle weakness, sensory impairment, and diminution or abolition of the ankle jerk. At higher levels, the knee jerk may be lost. The neurological disturbance is segmental in pattern, and is dependent on the level of the prolapse. Impulse symptoms are common. When the prolapse is large and central, the cauda equina may be affected, producing bladder disturbance and even paraplegia. Such an occurrence is a surgical emergency, and immediate exploration imperative.

When a disc prolapse occurs in the adolescent, there is striking restriction of movements in the lumbar spine. In the older patient, where degenerative changes have occurred in the annulus, symptoms may be produced by an extensive backward bulging of the disc without there being a frank localised annular tear.

Occasionally, in the young in particular, the nucleus may herniate (without an annular tear) into the substance of the vertebral bodies, giving rise to mild backache without root symptoms. This pattern of herniation (Schmorl's nodes) is diagnosed radiographically.

Apart from the large central prolapse all cases of acute disc prolapse are first treated by conservative methods. In the majority of cases symptoms subside with a two week period of strict bed rest on a firm bed. Analgesics are essential initially. If the response is good, the patient is then allowed up although he is warned to avoid lifting and bending in case of recurrence. In some centres spinal extension exercises may be advocated at this stage. If the response has only been moderate, a number of surgeons allow the patient to be ambulant after a POP jacket support has been applied. Alternatively, a corset support may be prescribed. If there is no response to two weeks' bed rest, the case must be carefully re-assessed before further treatment by bed rest is continued. Where there is ultimately an unsatisfactory response, or where residual symptoms are severe, myelography and exploration must be considered.

'Low back strain'

This condition is diagnosed by elimination: it is backache in which no obvious pathology, including prolapsed disc, can be found. It follows that although the condition is common and real enough, its cause is obscure and any description of pathology is pure conjecture. There are many synonyms for this syndrome: these include lumbago, lumbo-sacral strain, sprained back, lumbar fibrositis, lumbar myalgia, strained back ligaments, sacro-iliac strain and rheumatism. A number of cases diagnosed as suffering from this complaint develop at a later stage unequivocal signs of disc prolapse, and it may be that many are suffering from a minor disc lesion which has failed to produce the normal signs associated with that condition.

The patient is usually in the 20 to 45 age group, and complains of dull backache aggravated by activity. There may be a history of a minor injury, but usually no cause will be offered. Extensive radiation of pain is not a feature, and impulse symptoms do not occur. Physical signs are often slight; there is often a good if not full range of movements in the spine, and no neurological abnormality is detectable in the lower limbs.

Most cases respond to physiotherapy in the form of local heat and spinal extension exercises. In the older, resistant case a spinal support is often helpful. If symptoms are chronic, a change of employment to lighter work may have to be contemplated.

Coccydynia

In patients with this complaint of pain in the coccygeal area, there is often a history of a fall in the seated position on to a hard surface; consequently in a number of cases radiographs may reveal a fracture of the end piece of the sacrum, or show the coccyx to be subluxed into the anteverted position. Symptoms of pain on sitting and defaecation are often protracted for 6 to 12 months, but tend to resolve spontaneously. In stubborn cases conservative treatment should invariably be first employed (short-wave diathermy, ultrasound, injection of long acting local anaesthetics). If there is complete failure to respond to a long period of treatment, excision of the coccyx may be successful in relieving symptoms: early excision, however, carries a poor prognosis.

Low back pain

This is easily the commonest complaint of new patients attending orthopaedic clinics and the potential causes are legion; yet nearly all cases are found in the end to be suffering from the effects of a prolapsed intervertebral disc or from a 'low back strain'. It is important, however, that the rarer and often more serious causes of this common complaint are not overlooked; a logical systematic approach with these facts in mind is essential.

History. The following key points in the history should be determined.

1. Onset
   a. Was the onset insidious or sudden?
   b. What there a history of an injury such as for example a sudden twist or strain, or a sneeze in a flexed position?
   c. How long have symptoms been present?
   d. Is there claudication?

2. Previous history
   a. Is there a history of a previous similar attack?
   b. Is there a history of any other trouble with the spine?

3. Characteristics of the pain
   a. Where is the site of the maximal pain?
   b. Is there any radiation of pain into the limbs, and if so, what is its extent?
   c. Is the pain affected by coughing or sneezing? (impulse pain)
   d. Has the patient paraesthesiae in the limbs?
   e. Is the pain constant?
   f. What factors aggravate or improve the symptoms? (e.g. rest, activity, etc.)

At this stage, a history of a traumatic episode, sciatic radiation, paraesthesiae and impulse symptoms would be highly suggestive of a prolapsed intervertebral disc being the cause for the patient's symptoms.

Now history taking should swing to the patient's general health, and the other body systems. The following points should be made:

1. Is there any weight loss?
2. Is there a history of any abnormality in the gastro-intestinal system, with particular reference to the large bowel?
3. Are there any symptoms referable to the genito-urinary system, with particular reference to disturbance of micturition or menstruation?
4. Are there any pulmonary symptoms?

Any abnormality detected by these questions must be separately investigated and as a general rule it is wise to examine the abdomen, rectum and breasts routinely.

The spine should then be examined clinically, and if symptoms have remained unchanged over a two week period, radiological examination and estimation of the sedimentation rate should be carried out. At this stage any well defined spinal abnormality or disease should be detected, such as idiopathic scoliosis, Scheuermann's disease, senile kyphosis, ankylosing spondylitis, spondylolisthesis, tuberculous or pyogenic osteitis of the spine and osteo-arthritis. If these have been eliminated, the question whether symptoms are due to a prolapsed intervertebral disc should be considered. The history, clinical findings, and straight radiographs of the spine should be in harmony before it is reasonable to make this diagnosis. By elimination, the remaining substantial number of cases may be labelled as suffering from low-back strain, unless again there is an unusual feature of the history or examination suggesting caution or further examination or investigation.

Commoner causes of back complaints in the various age groups

Children
: TB in the spine
Scoliosis (especially congenital types)
Spondylolisthesis
Tumour
Calvé's disease

Adolescents
: Scheuermann's disease
Adolescent disc syndrome
Low back strain
Scoliosis (postural and idiopathic)
TB of the spine

Young adults
: Prolapsed intervertebral disc
Back strain
Ankylosing spondylitis
TB of the spine
Pyogenic osteitis of the spine
Coccydynia
Spinal stenosis

Middle-aged
: Prolapsed intervertebral disc
Back strain
Primary osteo-arthritis
Osteo-arthritis secondary to Scheuermann's disease, scoliosis, and old fracture
Spondylolisthesis
Pyogenic osteitis of the spine
Rheumatoid arthritis
Paget's disease
Coccydynia
Spinal stenosis

Elderly
: Osteo-arthritis
True senile kyphosis
Osteoporosis   } with or without fracture
Osteomalcia
Metastatic lesions in the spine

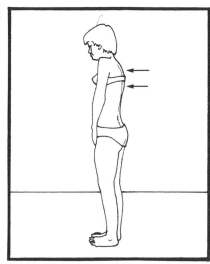

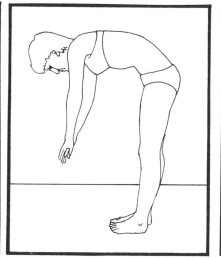

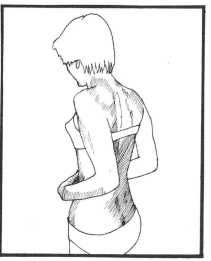

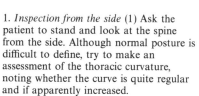

1. *Inspection from the side* (1) Ask the patient to stand and look at the spine from the side. Although normal posture is difficult to define, try to make an assessment of the thoracic curvature, noting whether the curve is quite regular and if apparently increased.

2. *Inspection* (2) It is valuable to know if the thoracic spine is mobile, especially if there is an increase in the curvature. Ask the patient to bend forwards carefully examining the flow of movement in the spine, and whether the curvature increases, demonstrating its mobility.

3. *Inspection* (3) Now ask the patient to stand upright, and brace back the shoulders to produce extension. An increased curvature (kyphosis) which is regular and mobile is found in postural kyphosis.

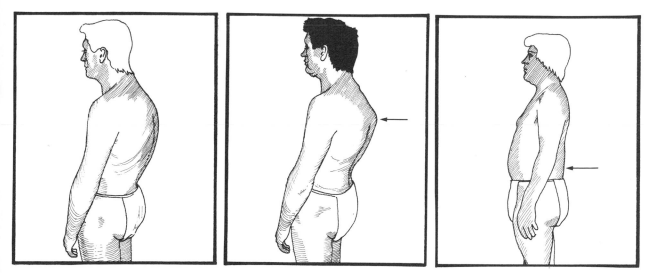

4. *Inspection* (4) If a regular, but fixed kyphosis is found, the commonest causes are senile kyphosis (sometimes with osteoporosis, osteomalcia or pathological fracture). Scheuermann's disease, and ankylosing spondylitis.

5. *Inspection* (5) If there is an angular kyphosis, with a gibbus or prominent vertebral spine, the commonest causes are fracture (traumatic or pathological) tuberculosis of the spine, or a congenital vertebral abnormality.

6. *Inspection* (6) Note the lumbar curvature. Flattening or reversal of the normal lumbar lordosis is a common finding in prolapsed intervertebral disc, osteoarthritis of the spine, infections of the vertebral bodies, and ankylosing spondylitis.

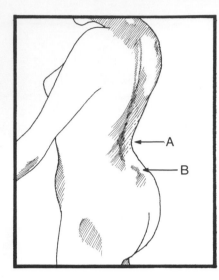

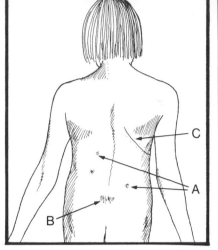

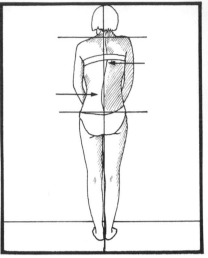

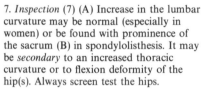

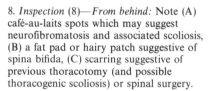

7. *Inspection* (7) (A) Increase in the lumbar curvature may be normal (especially in women) or be found with prominence of the sacrum (B) in spondylolisthesis. It may be *secondary* to an increased thoracic curvature or to flexion deformity of the hip(s). Always screen test the hips.

8. *Inspection* (8)—*From behind:* Note (A) café-au-laits spots which may suggest neurofibromatosis and associated scoliosis, (B) a fat pad or hairy patch suggestive of spina bifida, (C) scarring suggestive of previous thoracotomy (and possible thoracogenic scoliosis) or spinal surgery.

9. *Inspection* (9) Note the presence of any lateral curvature (scoliosis). The commonest scoliosis is a protective scoliosis in the lumbar region secondary to a PID. Note whether the shoulders and hips are level.

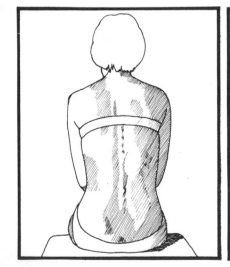

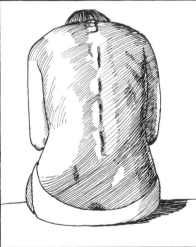

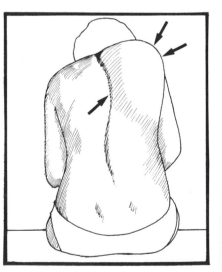

10. *Inspection* (10) In considering other causes of scoliosis, examine the spine with the patient sitting. Obliteration of an abnormal curve suggests that the scoliosis is mobile and secondary to shortening of a leg. Check relative leg lengths (see *Hip* 5).

11. *Inspection* (11) If on sitting the scoliosis persists, ask the patient to bend forwards. If the curve disappears, this suggests that it is quite mobile and most likely to be postural in origin.

12. *Inspection* (12) If the curvature remains, this suggests that the scoliosis is fixed (structural scoliosis). If a rib hump is present, this confirms the diagnosis.

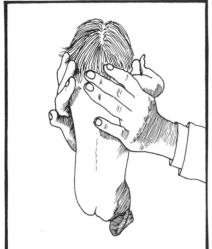

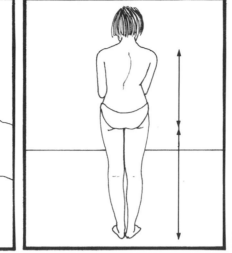

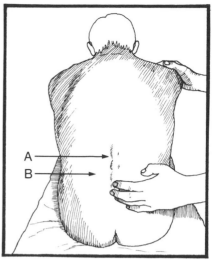

13. *Inspection* (13) In the case of infantile scoliosis, assess the ridigity of a curvature by noting any alterations as the child is lifted by the armpits.

14. *Inspection* (14) Note that where there is an idiopathic scoliosis with double fixed (primary) curves, the deformity may not be obvious on first inspection. There will however be shortening of stature with a trunk which is short in proportion to the limbs.

15. *Palpation* (1) Ask the patient to lean forwards if possible. Look for tenderness (A) between the spines of the lumbar vertebrae and lumbo-sacral junction (common in PID) and (B) over the lumbar muscles (common in PID and in low back strain).

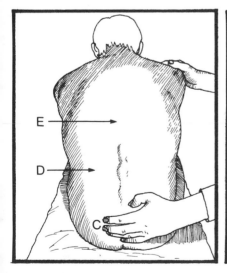

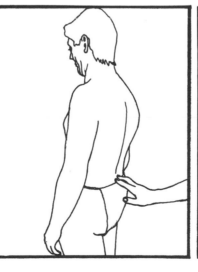

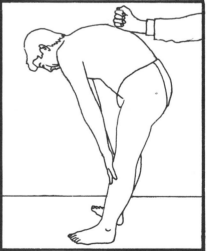

16. *Palpation* (2) Tenderness over the sacro-iliac joints (C) may occur in low back strain and in sacro-iliac joint infections. Re-examine with the patient prone. Renal tenderness (D) must be investigated fully. Look also for tenderness higher in the spine (E) e.g. from infection.

17. *Palpation* (3) With the patient standing, slide the fingers down the lumbar spine on to the sacrum. A palpable step at the lumbo-sacral junction is a feature of spondylolisthesis. Note any other curve irregularity (e.g. gibbus).

18. *Percussion:* Ask the patient to bend forwards. Lightly percuss the spine in an orderly progression from the root of the neck to the sacrum. Marked pain is a feature of tuberculous and other infections.

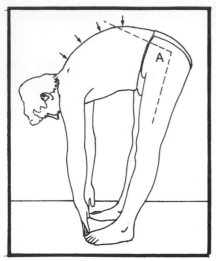

19. *Movements: Flexion* (1) Ask the patient to attempt to touch his toes while you closely watch the spine for smoothness of movement and any areas of restriction. Note that (A) hip flexion plays an important part, and can account for apparent motion in a rigid spine.

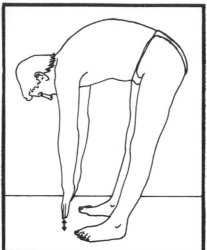

20. *Movements: Flexion* (2) Flexion may be recorded in several ways, the commonest being to note the distance between the fingers and the ground, e.g. 'the patient flexes to within 10 cm from the floor'. This is an indication of overall thoracic and lumbar movement, but ignores the hips.

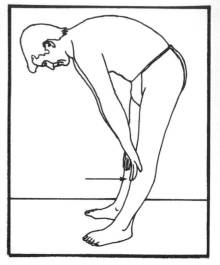

21. *Movements: Flexion* (3) Flexion may also be recorded 'the patient flexes so that the finger-tips reach mid-tibia — or other appropriate level. The majority of normal patients can reach the floor or within 7 cm from it. (Actual max. range flexion is approx. 45° thoracic, 60° lumbar.)

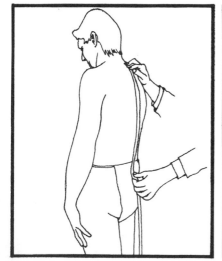

22. *Movements: Flexion* (4) For unequivocal evidence of mobility in the spine, first mark the spines of T1 and S1. Note that the spine of T1 is more conspicuous than that of C7, the so-called vertebra prominens. Measure the distance between these marks with the patient erect.

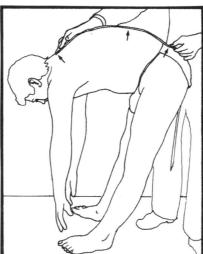

23. *Movements: Flexion* (5) Repeat with the spine fully flexed. The normal increase is about 10 cm in the adult. Gross reduction is an outstanding feature of ankylosing spondylitis. Movements in the thoracic and lumbar spine can be determined separately by marking and measuring from the spine of D12 in both directions.

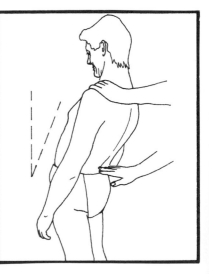

24. *Movements: Extension:* Ask the patient to arch his back, assisting him by steadying the pelvis and pulling back on the shoulder. Pain is common in PID. Accurate measurement is difficult. (Max. theoretical range thoracic 25°, lumbar 35°. Normal probably about 30° total.)

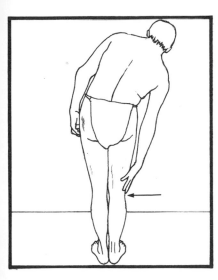

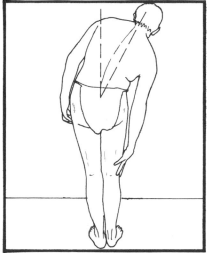

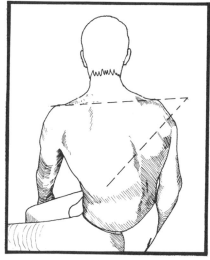

25. *Movements: Lateral flexion* (1) Ask the patient to slide the hands down the side of each leg in turn, and record the point reached, either in cm from the floor, or the position that the fingers reach in the legs.

26. *Movements: Lateral flexion* (2) Alternatively, measure the angle formed between a line drawn through T1, S1, and the vertical. The average range is 30° to either side, and the contributions of the thoracic and lumbar spine are usually equal.

27. *Movements: Rotation:* The patient should be seated, and be asked to twist round to each side. Rotation is measured between the plane of the shoulders and the pelvis. The normal maximum range is 40°, and is almost entirely *thoracic.* (Lumbar 5° or less.)

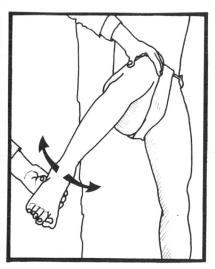

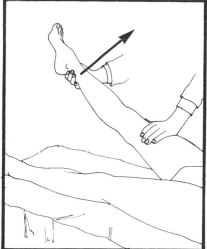

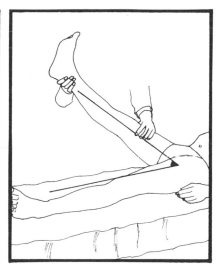

28. *Suspected PID:* Always start by screening the hips. O-A of the hip and PID are frequently confused. A full range of rotation in the hips with absence of pain at the extremes is generally all that is required to eliminate the former.

29. *Suspected PID: Straight leg raising test* (1) Assuming the hips are normal, raise the leg from the couch while watching the patient's face. Stop when the patient complains, and confirm that he is complaining of back or leg pain, and not hamstring tightness.

30. *Straight leg raising* (2) The result should be recorded as 'straight leg raising full' (no pain) or, e.g. 'SLR + ve on the right side at 60°'. Repeat on the other side. Make a separate note of the site of any pain the patient experiences. Back pain suggests central, and leg pain, lateral disc protrusion. Hamstring tightness is not significant.

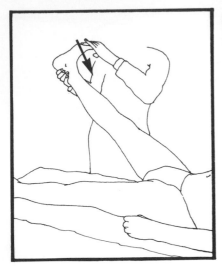

31. *Straight leg raising* (3) Passive dorsiflexion of the foot usually aggravates any pain, and this should be recorded. The SLR test is rarely negative in patients suffering from a PID (an exception is the high lumbar disc lesion) and is useful in assessing progress.

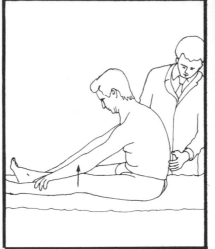

32. *Straight leg raising* (4) If there is some doubt regarding the severity of genuineness of the patient's complaints, ask him to sit up under the pretext of examining the back from behind. If symptoms are genuine and have an organic basis, it is unlikely that he will be capable of doing this without flexing his knees.

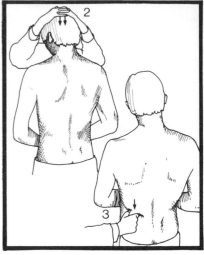

33. *Suspected PID: Functional overlay ctd:* (2) Apply pressure to the head. Overlay is suggested if this aggravates the back pain. (3) Pinch the skin at the sides. Such superficial stimulation should not produce deep-seated back pain. (4) Any motor or sensory disturbance should be segmental and localised. Widespread weakness and/or stocking anaesthesia also suggest overlay (but do carry out a thorough neurological and circulatory examination).

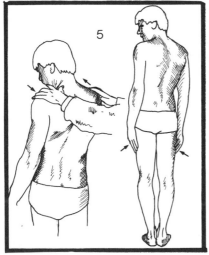

34. *Suspected PID: Functional overlay ctd:* (5) Note the amount of rotation required to produce pain in the back. Now ask the patient to keep his hands firmly at his side and repeat: the major part of the movement will now take place in the legs. Pain occurring with the same amount of apparent rotation again suggests overlay. In many centres, if three or more of the preceding tests are positive, surgery is considered to be contra-indicated.

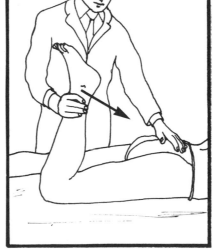

35. *Suspected PID: Reverse Lasegue test* (1) The patient should be prone. Flex each knee in turn. This gives rise to pain (by stretching of femoral nerve roots) in high lumbar disc lesions.

36. *Reverse Lasegue* (2) The pain produced in such a test if positive is normally aggravated by extension of the hip, and this should be noted. High disc lesions are rare compared with those affecting the L5-S1 and L4-L5 spaces.

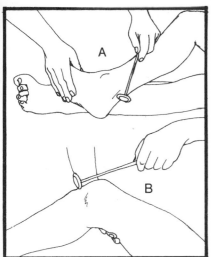

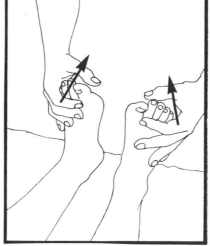

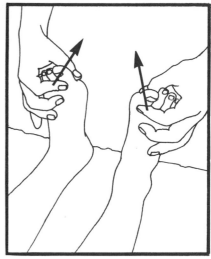

37. *Suspected PID ctd:* Look for further evidence of neurological involvement. A reduced or absent (A) ankle jerk (S1, 2) or (B) knee jerk (L3, 4) is a highly significant finding accompanying a positive straight leg raising or positive reverse Lasegue test.

38. *Suspected PID:* Root pressure from a disc may affect myotomes and dermatomes in a rather selective fashion (see *Segmental Innervation* section). Ask the patient to dorsiflex both feet. Now attempt to force them into plantar-flexion against his resistance (L45).

39. *Suspected PID:* Shift the grip to the great toes and test the power of dorsiflexion. Repeat with the lesser toes. (L4, 5). Now test the power of plantar-flexion of the great and lesser toes (S1, 2).

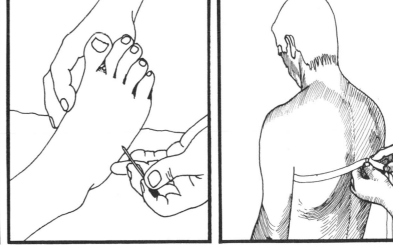

40. *Suspected PID:* Encircle the feet with the hands, and test the power of the peronei against the patient's resistance (L5, S1). Test the power of the quadriceps (L34) when a high disc lesion is suspected.

41. *Suspected PID:* Test sensation to pin prick in the dermatomes of the lower limb. Diminution of sensation at the side of the foot (S1) is one of the commonest findings (see also *Segmental and Peripheral Nerves of Lower Limb*).

42. *Suspected Ankylosing Spondylitis:* Always check the patient's chest expansion. This is often diminished at an early stage in the disease to less than 5 cm.

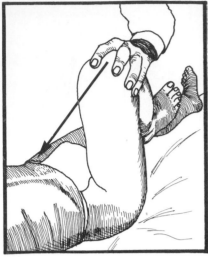

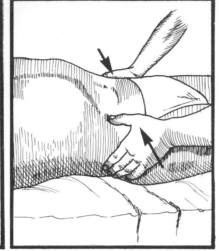

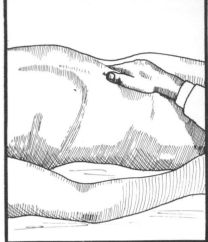

43. *Suspected sacro-iliac joint involvement* (1) Flex the hip and knee, and forcibly adduct the hip. Pain may accompany this manoeuvre in early ankylosing spondylitis, tuberculosis and other infections, and Reiter's syndrome, but many false positives do occur with this test.

44. *Suspected S-I joint involvement* (2) Note if pain is produced by pelvic compression (or by attempting to 'open out' the pelvis with the thumbs hooked round the anterior spines). True sacro-iliac joint pain may occur in women shortly before and after childbirth.

45. *Abdominal examination:* This is an essential part of the investigation of all cases of back pain, and where the history and other elements of the examination suggests, rectal or vaginal examination may also be necessary.

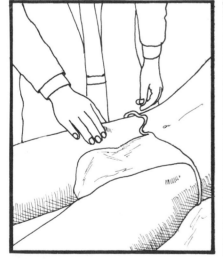

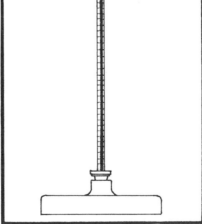

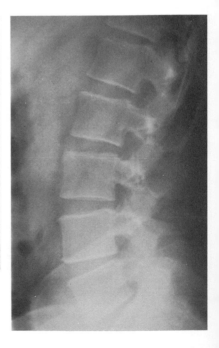

46. *Circulation:* The peripheral pulses and circulation should also be checked in all cases. Back and leg pain caused by arterial insufficiency are usually aggravated by activity, and absence of femoral pulsation is of particular significance.

47. *Sedimentation rate:* Estimation of the sedimentation rate is a valuable screening test in the investigation of all spinal-complaints. It is normal in PID, low back strain and Scheuermann's disease, but elevated in ankylosing spondylitis, many infections and neoplasms.

48. *Radiographs* (1) Normal lateral lumbar spine.

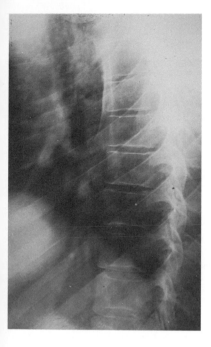

49. *Radiographs* (2) Normal lateral thoracic spine.

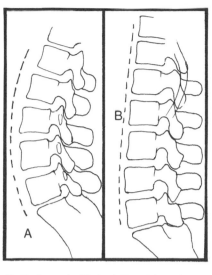

50. *Radiographs* (3) An A-P and lateral are the standard projections for both the lumbar and thoracic spine. Localised views of the lumbo-sacral junction are a useful addition. In the lateral note first the lumbar curve; (A) typical normal, (B) loss of lordosis (seen most often in PID).

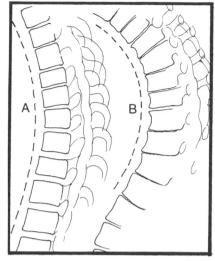

51. *Radiographs* (4) In the thoracic spine note (A) a typical normal curve, (B) an increased but regular curve typical of senile kyphosis. Scheuermann's disease is another frequent cause of a regular dorsal kyphosis.

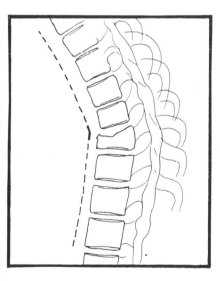

52. *Radiographs* (5) In both the lumbar and thoracic spine note any sharp alteration in the curvature, found typically where there is pathology restricted to one or two vertebral bodies, e.g. from fractures, TB or other infections, tumour, and osteomalacia with local collapse.

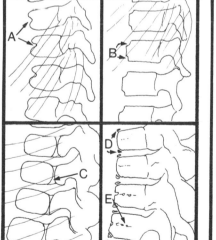

53. *Radiographs* (6) Now look at the shape of the bodies and the size of the discs. Compare with above and below. The following are normal in the child's spine. (A) Anterior clefts, (B) anterior notches, (C) incomplete fusion of elements, (D) epiphyses, (E) vascular tracks (which may persist).

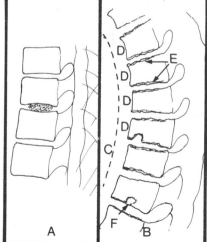

54. *Radiographs* (7) Note (A) disc calcification, (B) the typical appearance of Scheuermann's disease, with (C) kyphosis, (D) anterior wedging involving several vertebrae, (E) ragged appearance of the epiphyses. Note (F) central disc herniation (Schmorl's node) not necessarily associated.

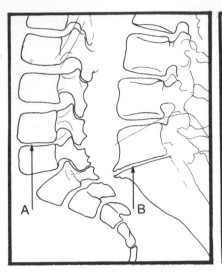

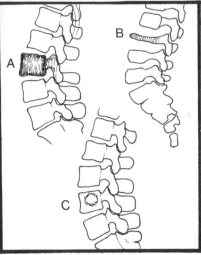

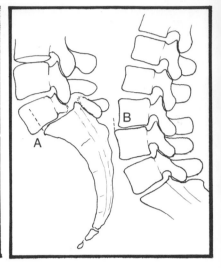

55. *Radiographs* (8) Note (A) disc narrowing at any level in the spine is the earliest evidence of TB and other infections. (B) Narrowing at L5-S1 and less commonly in the two spaces above occurs in long standing disc lesions (PID) and is often associated with ant. lipping.

56. *Radiographs* (9) Note (A) increased density and 'picture-frame' appearance of vertebrae seen in Paget's disease, (B) marked narrowing and density seen in Calve's disease (vertebra plana), (C) space occupying lesion in body usually due to tumour or infection (but note Schmorl's nodes).

57. *Radiographs* (10) Note the relationship of each vertebra to its neighbour. In particular note (A) spondylolisthesis (see also *Radiographs* 22), (B) retro-spondylolisthesis (usually associated with disc degeneration).

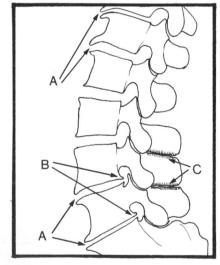

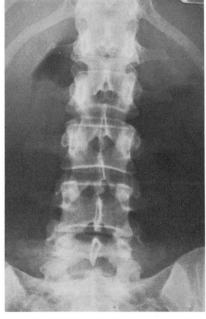

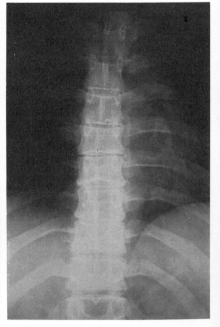

58. *Radiographs* (11) Lipping is seen in chronic disc lesions, mainly at L5–S1, but also at the other rarer disc prolapse sites. Note (A) anterior lipping, (B) posterior lipping. Lipping is also the main feature (at all levels) of O-A. Note (C) lumbar spine impingement.

59. *Radiographs* (12) Normal A-P view of the lumbar spine.

60. *Radiographs* (13) Normal A-P view of the thoracic spine.

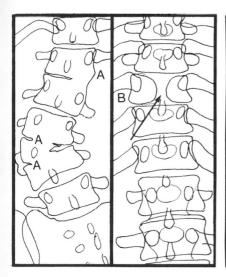

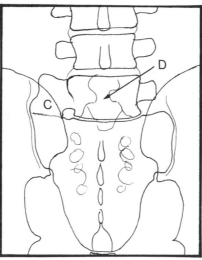

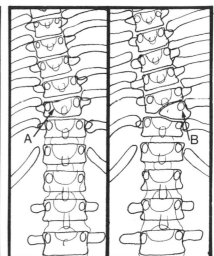

61. *Radiographs* (14) In the A-P view note the presence of any congenital abnormalities such as (A) congenital vertebral fusion, often associated with a congenital scoliosis, (B) anterior spina bifida in which there is failure of fusion of the vertebral body elements (usually symptom-free).

62. *Radiographs* (15) Note also any anomalies of the lumbo-sacral articulation such as (C) partial sacralisation of the fifth lumbar vertebra, a possible cause of low back pain. Note also (D) the presence of (posterior) spina bifida.

63. *Radiographs* (16) Note also the presence of any localised lateral angulation of the spine (A) due to lateral vertebral collapse e.g. from fracture, infection, tumour, osteoporosis or other causes. (B) Hemivertebra, a common cause of congenital scoliosis (note extra rib).

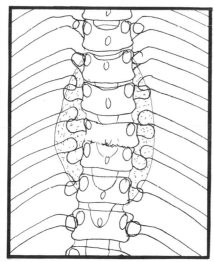

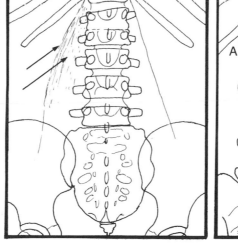

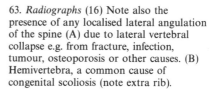

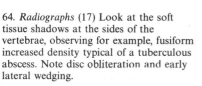

64. *Radiographs* (17) Look at the soft tissue shadows at the sides of the vertebrae, observing for example, fusiform increased density typical of a tuberculous abscess. Note disc obliteration and early lateral wedging.

65. *Radiographs* (18) Examine the psoas shadows for symmetry. Lateral displacement of the edge of the shadow, and increased density within the main area occupied by psoas suggests a psoas abscess, typically found in tuberculosis of the lumbar or lowermost thoracic spine.

66. *Radiographs* (19) Look for lateral lipping: (A) At D12–L1, it may be an early sign of ankylosing spondylitis, but there and elsewhere it usually indicates O-A. 'Bamboo spine' (B) is diagnostic of ankylosing spondylitis. Note body fusion and ligament calcification.

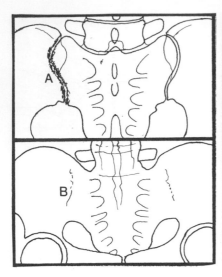

67. *Radiographs* (20) Look at the sacro-iliac joints. (A) Unilateral involvement (sclerosis, obliteration) may occur in TB and other infections. Any asymmetry should be investigated by oblique projections and if necessary, tomography. Bilateral involvement (B) is common in ankylosing spondylitis.

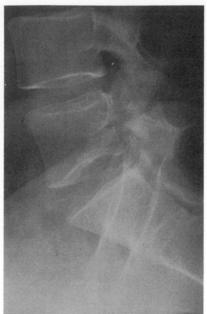

68. *Radiographs* (21) Normal localised lateral view of the lumbo-sacral junction.

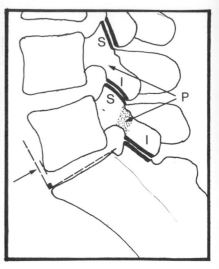

69. *Radiographs* (22) Look for evidence of spondylolisthesis. In the normal spine, the pars interarticularis (P) lying between (S) the superior and (I) the inferior articular facets is intact, and a vertical raised from the anterior margin of the sacrum lies in front of L5.

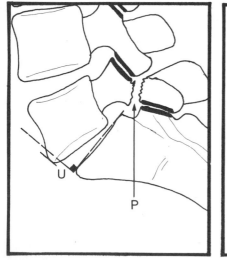

70. *Radiographs* (25) If spondylolisthesis is suspected, the lateral should always be taken with the patient standing. Note any defect (P) and forward slip (U). The deformity may occur between L5 and S1, and much less frequently between L4/L5 or L3/L4.

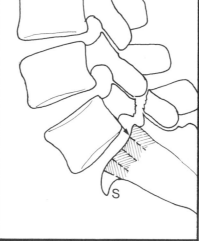

71. *Radiographs* (24) Note (S) New bone formation may make use of the anterior edge of the sacrum as a reference unreliable. Instead, note the relation of the posterior edge of the slipping vertebra to the one below. The example shows a forward slip of 25 per cent.

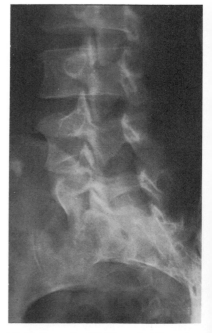

72. *Radiographs* (25) Normal oblique view of the lumbo-sacral junction.

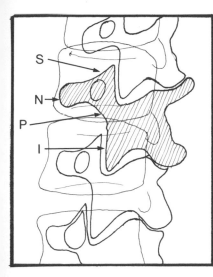

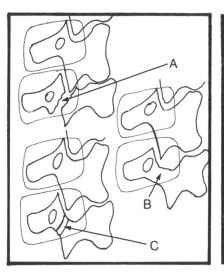

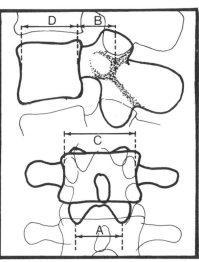

73. *Radiographs* (26) Oblique views are invaluable. In interpreting these, identify the 'Scotty dog' shadows. (N) The nose is formed by a transverse process, (S) the ear, by a superior articular process, (I) the front legs, by an inferior articular process, (P) the neck, by the pars interarticularis.

74. *Radiographs* (27) In spondylolisthesis (A) the 'dog' becomes decapitated due to forward slip and the inferior articular process of the vertebra above encroaches on the neck. In spondylolysis, where no slip has occurred, the neck (B) is elongated or (C) develops a collar.

75. *Radiographs* (28) Where spinal stenosis is suspected, calculate the canal to body ratio, AB:CD, where A = interpedicular distance, B = spinal canal front-to-back (measure to root of spinous process), C = width of vertebral body, D = body, front-to-back. The normal range is from approximately 1:2 to 1:4.5. Values greater than 4.5 suggest spinal stenosis, but other investigations (e.g. CAT scanning, myelography) may be indicated.

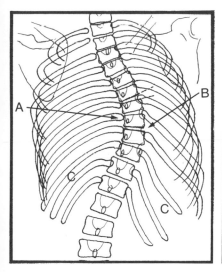

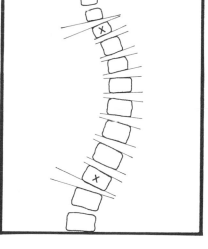

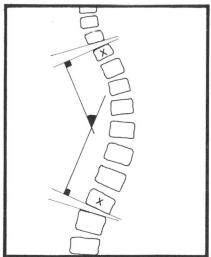

76. *Radiographs* (29) Note any structural scoliosis with (A) *on the concavity*, displacement of spines and narrowing of pedicles, (B) *on the convexity*, widening of disc spaces. (C) In the thorax, rib-cage distortion. Identify primary curves clinically or by lateral flexion radiographs.

77. *Radiographs* (30) In measuring the angular deformity (Cobb method), identify the limits of the primary curve by drawing tangents to the bodies and noting where the disc spaces begin to become widened on the concavity of the curve. The primary curve lies within these limits.

78. *Radiographs* (31) Now erect perpendiculars from the vertebrae which form the limits of the curve (marked 'X'). Note the angle between them which measures the primary curve, and which can be used for comparison with past and future radiographs. Kyphosis may be measured in a similar way.

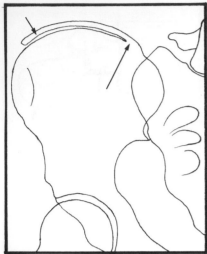

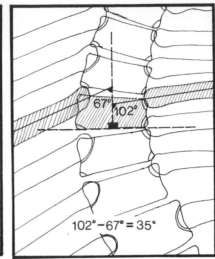

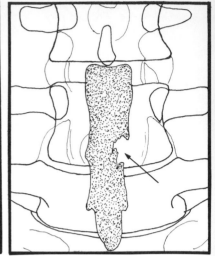

79. *Radiographs* (32) In late adolescence the appearance and progressing fusion of the iliac apophysis from behind forwards heralds skeletal maturity, and hence the time from which no further deterioration of a scoliotic curve should occur.

80. *Radiographs* (33) In *infantile scoliosis* note the difference in rib angles at the apex of the curve by the shown construction. A difference of 20° or more must be regarded as potentially progressive. An improvement over a three month period carries a good prognosis (Mehta).

81. *Radiographs* (34) *Myelography* is invaluable in confirming the presence and level of a PID or tumour.
Tomography is of particular value in the investigation of uncertain vertebral body lesions and of the SI joints.

8 Segmental and Peripheral Nerves of the Lower Limb

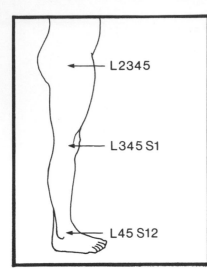

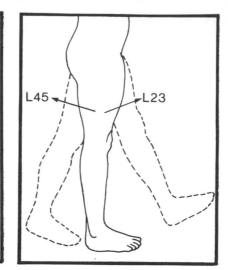

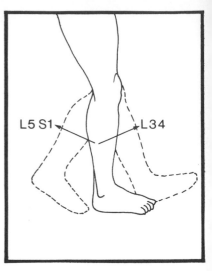

1. *Myotomes* (1) (see also *Segmental Distribution of Upper Limb*). Four consecutive spinal segments control each lower limb joint. The progression of control from hip to ankle is shown in the diagram.

2. *Myotomes* (2) Flexion of the hip (mainly ilio-psoas) is controlled by L2, 3. Extension of the hip (mainly gluteus maximus and the hamstrings) is controlled by L4, 5 (L2, 3 also control internal rotation, and L4, 5 external rotation of the hip.)

3. *Myotomes* (3) Extension of the knee and the knee jerk (quadriceps) is controlled by L3, 4. Flexion of the knee (mainly hamstrings) is controlled by L5, S1.

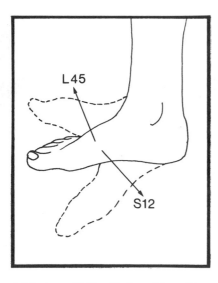

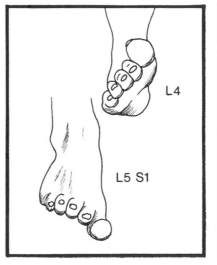

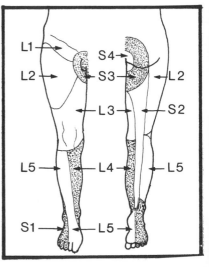

4. *Myotomes* (4) Dorsiflexion of the ankle is controlled by L4, 5 (mainly tibialis anterior and the long extensors of the hallux and toes). Plantar-flexion is controlled by S1, 2 (mainly the muscles of the calf). The same segments control the ankle jerk.

5. *Myotomes* (5) It is also useful to know that inversion (mainly tibialis anterior) is controlled by L4. Eversion is controlled by L5, S1 (the peronei).

6. *Dermatomes* Remember by the following: the side of the foot, S1, is commonly involved in L5–S1 disc lesions. L5 sweeps from the medial side of the foot next to S1 to the lateral side of the leg. L4 occupies the medial side, L2, 3 occupy the thigh. S3 supplies the 'bed-pan' area.

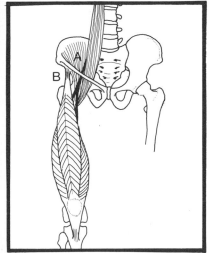

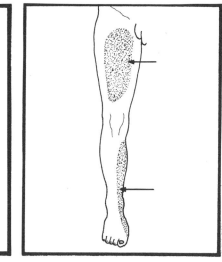

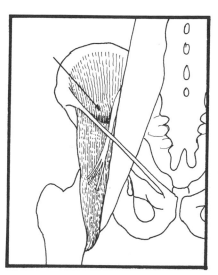

7. *Femoral Nerve L2, 3, 4* (1) *Motor distribution:* (A) Above the inguinal ligament the femoral nerve supplies ilio-psoas. (B) Below the inguinal ligament it supplies the quadriceps (also sartorius, pectineus).

8. *Femoral Nerve* (2) *Sensory distribution:* It supplies the front of the thigh, and through its terminal branch (the saphenous nerve) the medial side of the leg below the knee and the foot.

9. *Femoral Nerve* (3) *Sites of involvement:* Closed lesions of the femoral nerve are rare. Damage may occur when a haematoma is formed in the iliacus muscle causing local pressure. This is seen in haemophilia and in extension injuries of the hip.

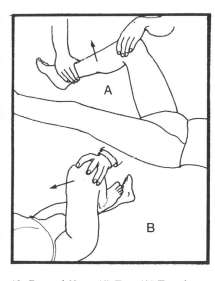

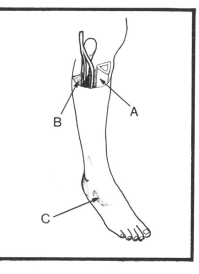

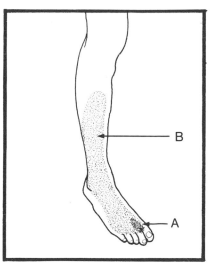

10. *Femoral Nerve* (4) *Test:* (A) Test the quadriceps by asking the patient to extend the knee against resistance. (B) Test the ilio-psoas (hip flexion against resistance). The response to these tests should determine the level. In doubtful cases try to elicit the knee jerk. Observe any quadriceps wasting, and test for loss of sensation to pin prick in the area supplied by the nerve.

11. *Common Peroneal Nerve L45S12: Motor distribution:* (A) Muscles of the anterior compartment (tib. anterior, ext. hallucis longus, ext. dig. longus, peroneus tertius). (B) Muscles of peroneal compartment (peroneus brevis and longus). (C) On the foot, extensor dig. brevis.

12. *Common Peroneal Nerve* (2) *Sensory distribution:* (A) First web space (deep peroneal contribution). (B) Dorsum of foot and front and side of leg (superficial peroneal contribution).

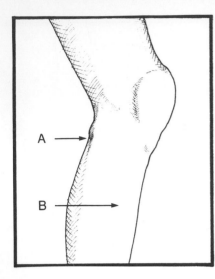

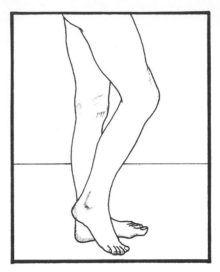

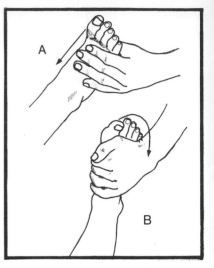

13. *Common Peroneal* (3) *Sites:* (A) Fibular neck — e.g. *Trauma* (lateral ligament injuries of the knee, direct blows, pressure from plaster casts or the side irons of a Thomas splint), *Ganglion, Ischaemia* (e.g. tourniquet) and many neurological disorders. (B) The deep peroneal branch in anterior compartment syndrome.

14. *Common Peroneal Nerve* (4) *Deformity:* The patient will have a drop foot, and there will be disturbance of the gait; either the leg will be lifted high to allow the plantar flexed foot to clear the ground, or the foot will be slid along the ground with rapid wear of the shoe.

15. *Common Peroneal Nerve* (5) (A) Ask the patient to dorsiflex the foot (deep peroneal branch) and (B) to evert the foot (superficial peroneal branch). Test for sensation in the area of distribution of the nerve. Note any wasting of the front or side of the leg.

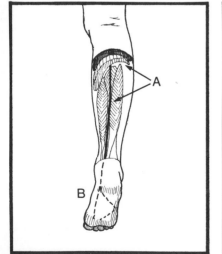

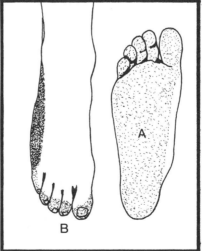

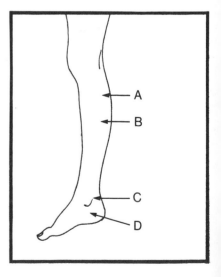

16. *Posterior Tibial Nerve: L45 S123: Motor distribution:* (A) Soleus and deep muscles of the posterior compartment (tibialis posterior, flexor hallucis longus, flexor digitorum longus). (B) All the muscles of the sole of the foot through the medial and lateral plantar nerves.

17. *Post. Tibial* (2) *Sensory distribution:* (A) Sole of foot through the medial and lateral plantar nerves whose territory includes (B) the nail beds and distal phalanges. Note that the side of the foot is supplied by the sural nerve derived from the medial popliteal and common peroneal.

18. *Post Tibial* (3) *Common sites of involvement:* (A) When passing under the soleal arch, from tibial fractures. (B) Ischaemic lesions of calf (post, compartment syndrome tight plasters), and diabetic neuropathy. (C) Behind medial malleolus (lacerations and fractures). (D) In tarsal tunnel syndrome.

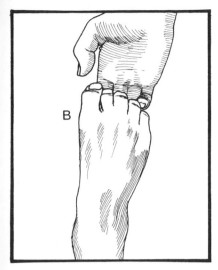

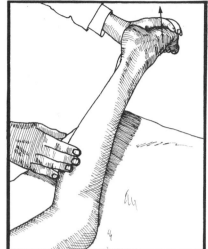

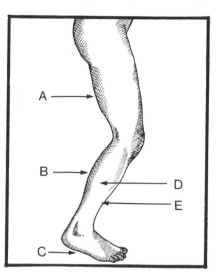

19. *Post. Tibial* (4) *Diagnosis:* Note any muscle wasting in the sole of the foot, clawing of the toes and trophic ulceration. (B) Test the power of toe flexion. (C) Look for sensory loss in the area supplied by the nerve.

20. *Medial Popliteal Nerve: L45 S123:* The nerve is seldom injured as it is deeply situated. The findings are essentially the same as in lesions of the posterior tibial nerve, but with wasting and loss of power of plantar-flexion due to paralysis of gastrocnemius as well as soleus.

21. *Sciatic Nerve: L45 S123: Motor distribution:* (A) The hamstrings in the thigh. (B) The superficial and deep muscles of the calf by the medial popliteal and the posterior tibial. (C) The sole muscles by the medial and lateral plantar nerves. (D) The peronei by the superficial peroneal. (E) The anterior compartment by the deep peroneal.

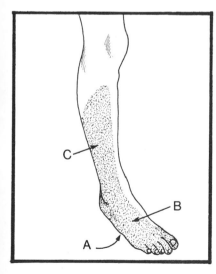

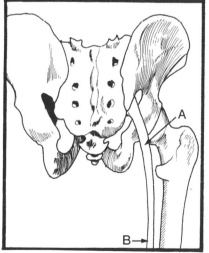

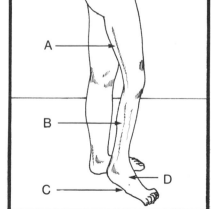

22. *Sciatic Nerve* (2) *Sensory distribution:* (A) The entire sole. (B) The dorsum of the foot. (C) The lateral aspect of the leg and lateral half of the calf. The medial side of the calf and foot are spared. If the posterior cutaneous nerve of the thigh is involved, there is loss sensation at the back of the thigh.

23. *Sciatic Nerve* (3) *Sites involved:* (A) Behind the hip, e.g. after posterior dislocation of the hip, after some pelvic fractures (rare) and after hip surgery. (B) Following deep wounds back of thigh (also uncommon). Do not confuse with root involvement in intervertebral disc prolapse.

24. *Sciatic Nerve* (4) *Diagnosis:* Note extensive wasting, (A) thigh, (B) calf and peronei, (C) sole of foot. Note (D) drop foot. Observe any trophic ulceration. Note loss of power in the hamstrings and all three compartments below the knee, absent ankle jerk and extensive sensory loss.

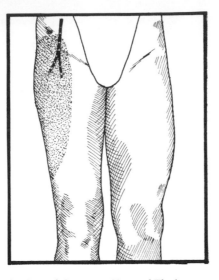

25. *Lateral Cutaneous Nerve of Thigh (L23):* The nerve pierces the lateral portion of the inguinal ligament and supplies the lateral aspect of the thigh. It may be compressed as it passes through the inguinal ligament, giving pain and paraesthesiae in the leg (meralgia paraesthetica).

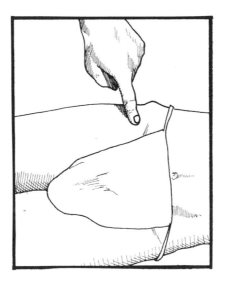

26. *Lateral Cutaneous Nerve of Thigh:* (2) *Test:* Pressure over the nerve may give rise to paraesthesiae in the thigh. Test for sensory impairment in the area supplied by the nerve.

9 The Hip

Congenital dislocation of the hip

Congenital dislocation of the hip is a condition in which one or both hips are dislocated at birth, or dislocate in the first few weeks of life. It is much commoner in girls than boys; there is a familial tendency, and a well established geographical distribution of the disorder. It may occur in conjunction with other congenital defects.

CDH in the neonate

All newly born children should have a routine examination of the hips which should disclose the presence of a frank dislocation or instability in the hip. Particular care should be taken over the initial examination when there is a family history of this condition. Ideally too, all hips should be re-examined at six months before weight bearing commences. Although a number of children with instability may recover without treatment, it is not possible to differentiate these from those who will progress to full dislocation. In the routine management of this problem, all children with dislocation or instability are therefore treated by splintage of the hips in abduction using a simple padded metal splint (Malmo or van Rosen splint, Barlow splint). Splintage should be instituted without delay, and after 12 weeks stability is achieved in the majority of cases. When stability has been obtained, the splint can be discarded, but the child must remain under surveillance in order to detect the rare but occasional late secondary dislocation.

CDH in the older child

It is now uncommon for a child to be seen for the first time with congenital dislocation of the hip after weight-bearing has commenced, although this was routine in the past before the standard screening of newly born children became established. The later the age of presentation the more formidable are the problems of treatment, so that any child who is seen with a disturbance of gait or posture, shortening of a limb, or complaint of the hip must be most carefully examined to exclude this condition. If dislocation is diagnosed late, the aims of treatment are as follows:

1. The head of the femur, if displaced proximally, must be brought down to the level of the acetabulum (usually by a short period of traction).

103

2. The head of the femur must be reduced into the acetabulum. In many cases this may be achieved by rotation of the hips, but sometimes surgery is required to remove an inturned obstructing labrum (excision of limbus).

3. The head of the femur must be maintained in concentricity with the acetabulum to stimulate healthy growth of both fermoral head and acetabulum. Where a good acetabulum is present, plaster fixation for a prolonged period may suffice. Where the acetabulum is shallow or sloping, it may be necessary to rotate the acetabulur plane into a more horizontal position (e.g. by a Salter or pelvic osteotomy).

4. Where there is marked anteversion of the femoral head, this may have to be corrected by a de-rotational osteotomy of the femur.

CDH in the adult

Where treatment in childhood has been unsuccessful, or even where the condition has not been diagnosed, a patient may seek help during the third and fourth decades of life. Symptoms may arise from the hips or the spine. In the hips, secondary arthritic changes occur in the false joint which may form between the dislocated femoral head and the ilium with which it comes in contact. In the spine, osteo-arthritic changes are a result of long standing scoliosis (in the unilateral case) or increased lumbar lordosis (in both unilateral and bilateral cases). In a few cases hip replacement surgery may be considered, otherwise the treatment follows the lines of conservative management of osteo-arthritis of the hips and spine.

The dysplastic hip

Hip dysplasia is a condition in which one of the principal features is that the femoral head is imperfectly contained by the acetabulum. The acetabular slope is frequently greater than normal, so that the central area only of the femoral head transmits the forces of weight-bearing to the acetabulum. This predisposes the hip to osteo-arthritis and in some cases instability. The symptoms are those of osteo-arthritis of the hip, and they may present during the second and third decades of life. Rapid deterioration is the rule. In the younger patient, a Chiari osteotomy of the pelvis, an acetabular shelf operation or a high femoral osteotomy may improve the containment of the femoral head, relieve symptoms, and slow the onset of osteo-arthritis. In the older patient, replacement arthroplasty may be considered.

The irritable hip

In childhood there are a number of conditions affecting the hip which are indistinguishable in their initial stages. They all give rise to a limp, restriction of movements, and sometimes pain in the joint (irritable hip). Children with this history are admitted routinely and treated by light traction until a firm diagnosis has been made. The commonest conditions responsible for irritable hip are transient synovitis, Perthes' disease, and tuberculosis of the hip.

Transient synovitis. This is the commonest cause of the irritable hip. The child presents with a limp, and there is sometimes a history of preceding minor trauma which in some cases at least is coincidental. There is restriction of extension and internal rotation in the affected joint, but there is no systemic upset and the sedimentation rate is generally normal. Radiographs of the hip sometime give confirmatory evidence of synovitis, but no other pathology is demonstrable. Aspiration and culture of synovial, fluid (which is not routinely performed) fail to provide any evidence of infection. A full recovery after three to six weeks' bed rest is the rule.

Perthes' disease. In this condition there is a disturbance of the blood supply to the epiphysis of the femoral head so that a variably sized portion undergoes a form of avascular necrosis. The cause is unknown. It is commoner in boys than girls, and one or both hips may be involved; when both hips are affected, they may be involved simultaneously or with an interval between them. Vague pain in the region of the hips, thighs or knees is a frequent accompaniment. As a rule, radiographic changes are well established by the time the child presents with symptoms, and the diagnosis is made on these findings; clinically it may be suspected by the history, the child's age and sex, and by the restriction of rotation in the affected hip.

The prognosis is dependent on the position and extent of the area of the femoral head involved. When a large part of the epiphysis is affected, there is a tendency to flattening of the femoral head which is mirrored by the acetabulum, predisposing the hip to osteo-arthritis later in life.

Where pain is present the hip is treated by bed rest, preferably with leg traction. From the initial or serial radiographs it is often possible to identify those hips which carry a good prognosis, and where active treatment is neither of value nor required. The results of intervention in the cases which carry a poor prognosis are perhaps less clear. The lines of treatment frequently advocated aim either at reducing weight-bearing deformation of the head (by bed rest, a Snyder sling or calliper) or by improving head/acetabular congruity by osteotomy.

Tuberculosis. Tuberculosis of the hip is now rare in Britain. The child walks with a limp and often complains of pain in the groin or knee. Night pain is a feature. Rotation in the hip becomes limited, a fixed flexion deformity develops, and muscle wasting occurs. Radiographs of the hip in the early stages shown rarefaction of bone in the region of the hip and widening of the joint space. As the disease advances, there is progressive joint destruction with abscess formation and sometimes dislocation. The diagnosis is usually confirmed by histological and bacteriological examination of synovial biopsy specimens, or by bacteriological examination of the aspirate.

In early cases complete resolution may be hoped for by anti-tuberculous therapy, bed rest and traction. In the advanced case, joint debridement is carried out with efforts to obtain a bony fusion of the joint.

Acute pyogenic arthritis of the hip

The *Staphyloccocus* in the organism most frequently responsible for acute infections in the hip joint. The infection is blood borne, and diagnosis is seldom difficult. The onset is rapid, with high fever and toxaemia. All movements of the hip are severely impaired and accompanied by great pain and protective muscle spasm. The organism responsible may be isolated by blood culture or joint aspiration. Treatment is by use of the appropriate antibiotic in large doses to obtain a high local concentration. Bed rest and immobilisation are also essential.

Slipped femoral epiphysis

This is a disease of adolescence and is commoner in boys than girls. The attachment of the femoral epiphysis to the femoral neck loosens, so that the head appears to slide downwards on the femoral neck, giving rise eventually to a coxa vara deformity of the hip. The cause is unknown. In a number of cases there is a history of preceding trauma. A striking feature, however, is that in a high proportion of cases there is evidence of a hormonal disturbance. Many are fat, having the appearance of those suffering from the Fröhlich syndrome.

Pain may occur in the groin or knee, and if the onset is very acute, weight-bearing may become impossible. There is usually restriction of internal rotation and abduction in the hip. The diagnosis is confirmed radiographically, the earliest changes being seen in the lateral projections.

Slight degrees of slip are treated by internal fixation of the epiphysis without reduction. If there is a large amount of acute displacement, reduction may be attempted before fixation. If the slip is long standing, osteotomy of the femoral neck (to correct the deformity) may be preferable to attempted reduction if the risks of avascular necrosis are to be avoided. During convalescence from surgery the other hip should be kept under surveillance in case it becomes symptomlessly involved.

Primary osteo-arthritis of the hip

Primary osteo-arthritis of the hip occurs in the middle-aged and elderly, and is often associated with overweight and overwork, although in many cases no obvious cause may be found.

Pain is often illocalised in the hip, groin, buttock or trochanter, and may be referred to the knee. Sleep is often disturbed and the general health of the patient becomes undermined as a result. Stiffness may declare itself in difficulty in putting on stockings and cutting the toe nails.

Fixed flexion and adduction contractures are common, with apparent shortening of the affected limb. In the early stages weight reduction, physiotherapy and analgesics may be helpful; total hip replacement is the treatment of choice in the advanced stage.

Secondary osteo-arthritis of the hip

The symptoms of secondary osteo-arthritis of the hip are identical to those of primary osteo-arthritis. The condition occurs most frequently as a sequel to congenital dislocation of the hip, congenital coxa vara, hip dysplasia, Perthes' disease, tuberculous or pyogenic infections, slipped femoral epiphysis, and avascular necrosis secondary to femoral neck fracture or traumatic dislocation of the hip.

In secondary osteo-arthritis, a younger age group is generally involved than in the case of primary osteo-arthritis. In the unilateral case hip fusion must be considered as an alternative to replacement arthroplasty, especially where there has been a history of preceding infection. Where pain is more a problem than stiffness, MacMurray's osteotomy of the hip may sometimes be of value.

Rheumatoid arthritis

The hip joints are frequently involved in rheumatoid arthritis. When both hips and knees are affected, the disability may be profound. In the well selected case replacement of one or both hips may give a striking improvement in the patient's symptoms and mobility.

Other conditions affecting the hip

Of the rarer conditions affecting the hip joint, the following are not infrequently overlooked.

1. Ankylosing spondylitis may present as pain and stiffness in the hip in a young man. There may be no complaint of back pain, but there is almost invariably radiographic evidence of sacro-iliac joint involvement.

2. Reiter's syndrome may also first present in the hip.

3. Primary bone tumours are uncommon; of these, osteoid osteoma involving the femoral neck may be a cause of persistent hip pain. As this tumour is always small, repeated radiographic examination with well exposed films may be required to show it.

The following important points should always be remembered in dealing with the hip joint:

1. *The commonest cause of hip pain in the adult is pain referred from a prolapsed intervertebral disc. Hip movements are not impaired,* and there are almost invariably signs of the primary pathology, e.g. diminution of straight leg raising.

2. *In the elderly, pain in the hip with inability to weight bear is frequently due to a fracture of the femoral neck or of the pubic rami.* In an appreciable number of cases there is no history of injury, and radiographic examination is essential.

3. *Flexion contracture of the hip may result from psoas spasm secondary to inflammation or pus in the region of its sheath in the pelvis.* This is seen for example in appendicitis, appendix abscess or other pelvic inflammatory disease. Examination of the abdomen is essential.

Approximate Age Distribution of the Main Causes of Hip Symptoms

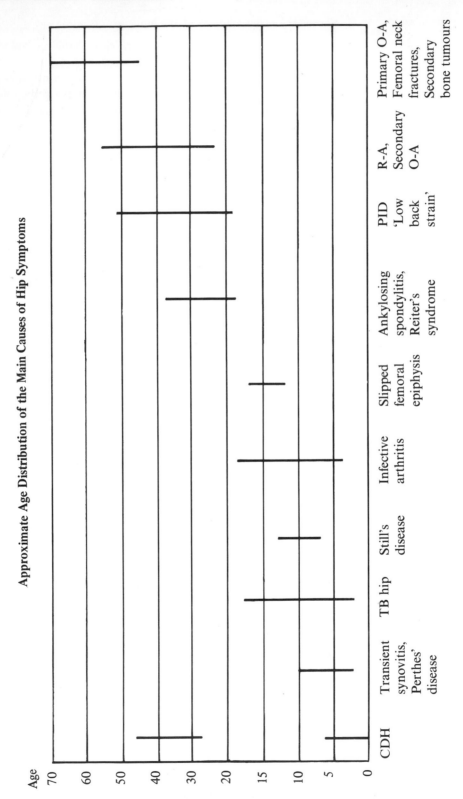

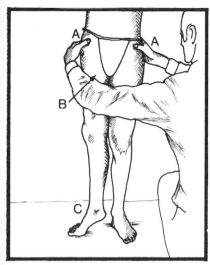

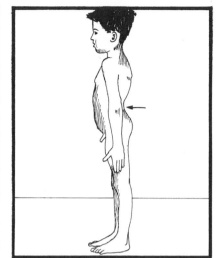

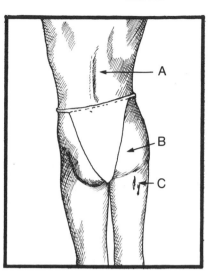

1. *Inspection:* (1) Examine the standing patient from the front. Note (A) any pelvic tilting (e.g. from adduction or abduction deformity of the hip, short leg, scoliosis), (B) muscle wasting (e.g. secondary to infection, disuse, polio), (C) rotational deformity (common in osteo-arthritis).

2. *Inspection:* (2) Examine the patient from the side. Note any increased lumbar lordosis suggestive of fixed flexion deformity of the hip(s).

3. *Inspection:* (3) Look at the patient from behind. Note (A) any scoliosis (possibly secondary to pelvic tilting, from for example an adduction deformity of the hip), (B) gluteal muscle wasting (e.g. from disuse, infection), (C) sinus scars (e.g. secondary to tuberculosis).

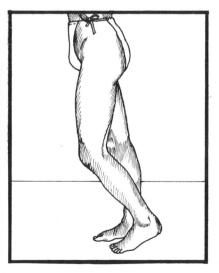

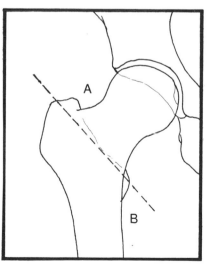

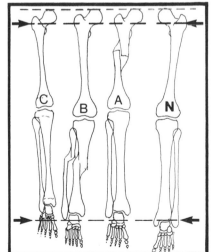

4. *Gait:* Observe the gait from the front, side and behind. Analysis is often difficult but grows from experience. In particular try to assess the stride and dwell time on each side, and the possible factors of pain, stiffness, shortening, and gluteal insufficiency.

5. *Shortening* (1) It is important in the examination of the hip and the lower limb to determine the presence or abscense of shortening. In *true shortening*, the affected limb is physically shorter than the other. This may be caused by pathology (A) above or proximal to the greater trochanter or (B) distal to the trochanters.

6. *True shortening:* (2) True shortening from causes distal to the trochanters most frequently results from (A) old fractures of the femur or (B) of tibia, (C) growth disturbance (e.g. from polio, bone or joint infection or epiphyseal trauma). (N) Normal side for comparison.

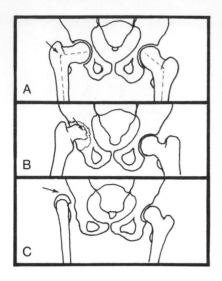

7. *True shortening* (3) *Above the trochanter* causes include (A) coxa vara (e.g. from neck fractures, slipped epiphysis, Perthes' disease, congenital coxa vara, (B) loss of articular cartilage (from infection, arthritis), (C) dislocation of the hip.

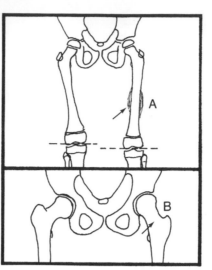

8. *Shortening* (4) Very rarely *lengthening of the other limb* gives relative true shortening. This may be due to (A) stimulation of bone growth from increased vascularity (e.g. after long bone fracture in children, or bone tumour), (B) coxa valga (e.g. following polio).

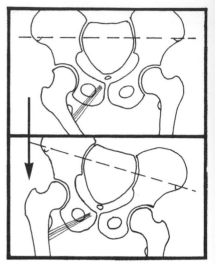

9. *Shortening* (5) In apparent shortening the limb is not altered in length, but appears short as a result of an adduction contracture of the hip which has to be compensated for by tilting of the pelvis.

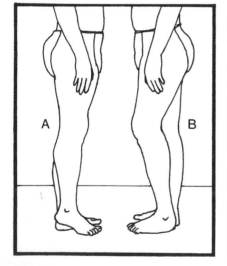

10. *Shortening* (6) Limb shortening may be compensated by (A) plantar-flexion of the foot on the affected side or by (B) flexion of the knee on the other or (C) by pelvic tilting which in turn may be compensated by the development of a lumbar scoliosis.

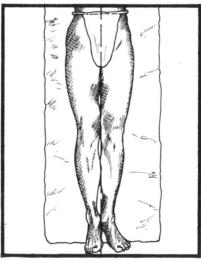

11. *Shortening: Examination* (1) The patient should be adjusted to lie squarely on the couch, with the trunk and legs parallel to its edge. The position of the pelvis should be observed (by the position of the anterior superior iliac spines) and adjusted where possible.

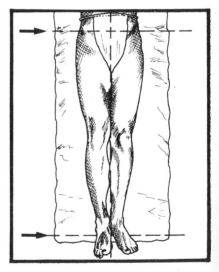

12. *Shortening: Examination* (2) In the normal patient the heels should be level, and the plane of the spines at right angles to the edge of the couch.

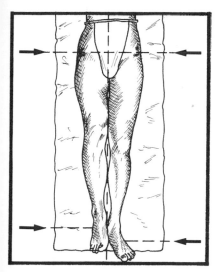

13. *Shortening: Examination* (3) Where there is significant true shortening, the heels will not be level (the discrepancy is a guide to the amount of shortening) and the pelvis will not be tilted. The site and amount of shortening must now be further investigated.

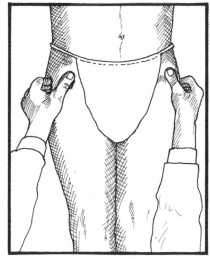

14. *Shortening: Examination* (4) Begin by hooking the thumbs under the anterior spines. Feel for the greater trochanters with the fingers. If the distance between the thumb and fingers is shorter on one side, this suggests that the pathology lies above the trochanters.

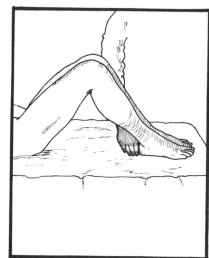

15. *Shortening: Examination* (5) If in the last test there was no evidence of shortening above the trochanter, look for causes below the trochanter. Slightly flex both knees and hips, and place a hand behind the heels to check that you now have them squarely together.

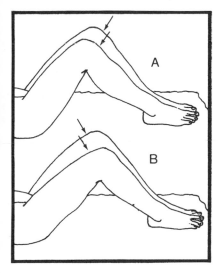

16. *Shortening: Examination* (6) The position of the two knees should be compared. (A) This appearance suggests femoral shortening. (B) This appearance is suggestive of tibial shortening.

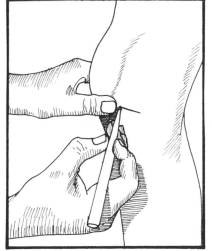

17. *Shortening: Examination* (7) Further confirmation of tibial shortening may be made by direct measurement. Flex the knees and mark the line of the knee joint.

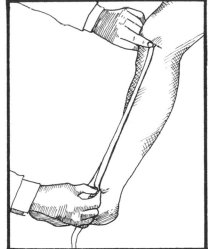

18. *Shortening: Examination* (8) Now measure from the mark to the tip of the medial malleolus. Compare the two sides. Any difference indicates true tibial shortening. Note also any obvious tibial irregularity suggestive of old fracture.

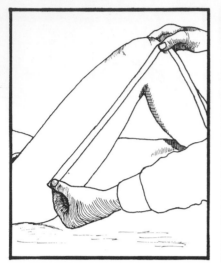

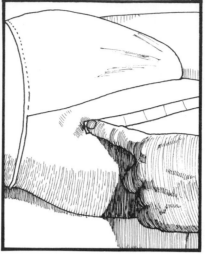

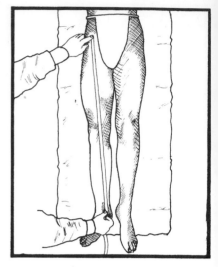

19. *Shortening: Examination* (9) Measurement of femoral shaft shortening can only be attempted in the thin patient where the tip of the greater trochanter is easily palpable. Measure from the trochanter to the lateral joint line and compare the sides.

20. *Shortening: Examination* (10) Measurement of total (true) leg shortening is the most valuable single assessment, although it gives itself no indication of site. Place the metal end of the tape over the anterior spine and press it backwards until it hooks under its inferior edge.

21. *Shortening: Examination* (11) Now measure to the middle or inferior border of the medial malleolus. Compare the sides, and always repeat the measurements until consistency is obtained. Deformity of the pelvis (which is rare) may sometimes lead to errors in assessment.

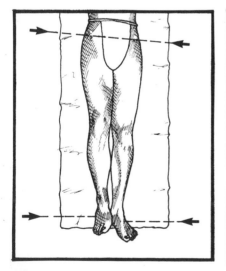

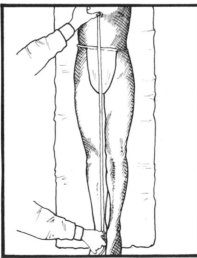

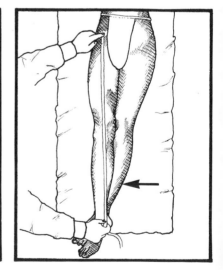

22. *Shortening: Examination* (12) Pelvic tilting which is uncorrectable, with heel discrepancy indicates apparent shortening of the limb. It may of course be accompanied by some true shortening. The discrepancy at the heels is a measure of its degree.

23. *Shortening: Examination* (13) Apparent shortening may also be assessed by comparing the distances between the xiphisternum and each medial malleolus.

24. *Shortening: Examination* (14) When there is an adduction deformity of the hip, and the leg lengths are being measured to assess any accompanying true shortening, the good leg should be adducted by the same amount before commencing measurement between the anterior spines and malleoli.

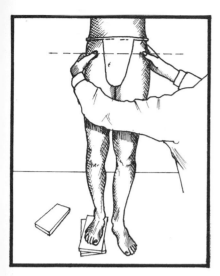

25. *Shortening: Examination* (15) True leg shortening may also be measured by blocking up the short leg until the pelvis is level.

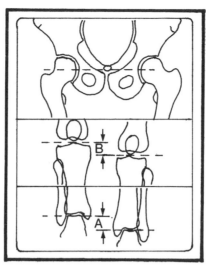

26. *Shortening: Examination* (16) In the difficult case, sequential radiographs of the hips, knees and ankles, taken on a single plate without moving the patient afford accurate comparison of the sides. For example, (A) indicates overall shortening, (B) indicates femoral shortening.

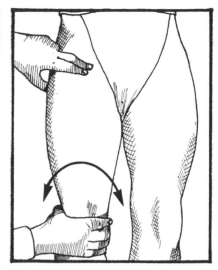

27. *Palpation* (1) Place the fingers over the head of the femur below the inguinal ligament, lateral to the femoral artery. Note any tenderness. Now rotate the leg medially and laterally. Crepitations arising in the hip joint may be detected in this way.

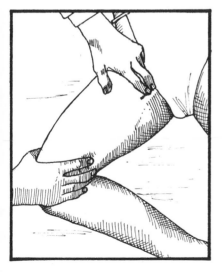

28. *Palpation* (2) Palpate the origin of adductor longus. Tenderness occurs here in sports injuries (strain of adductor longus) and in patients developing adductor contractures in osteo-arthritis of the hip.

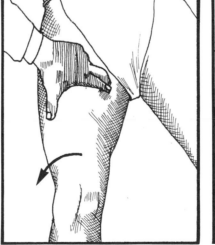

29. *Palpation* (3) Externally rotate the leg and palpate the lesser trochanter. Tenderness occurs here in strains of the ilio-psoas as a result of athletic injuries.

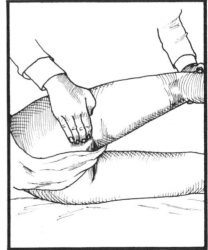

30. *Palpation* (4) Palpate the region of the ischial tuberosity looking for tenderness. Strain of the hamstring origin occurs as a result of athletic activities, especially in children. Less commonly athletic injuries may affect the anterior superior and inferior spines.

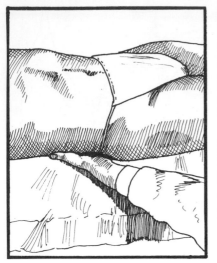

31. *Movements: Extension* (1) Place a hand behind the lumbar spine so that you may assess its position.

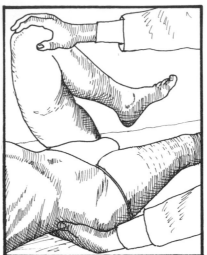

32. *Movements: Extension* (2) Now flex the *good* hip fully, observing with the hand that the lumbar curvature is fully obliterated.

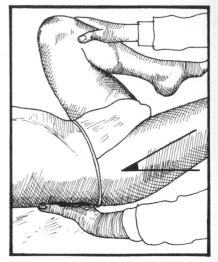

33. *Movements: Extension* (3) If the hip being examined rises from the couch, this indicates *loss of extension in that hip* (also described as *fixed flexion deformity of the hip*). Any loss should be measured and recorded. This test is usually referred to as Thomas's test.

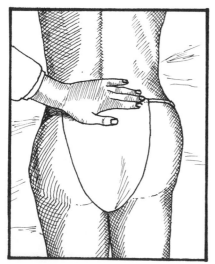

34. *Movements: Extension* (4) To check smaller losses of extension, especially when the other hip is normal, turn the patient over on to his face and steady the pelvis with one hand.

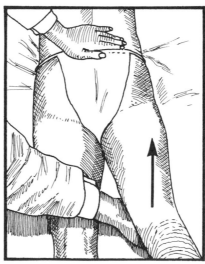

35. *Movements: Extension* (5) Lift each leg and compare the range.
Normal range = 5–20°
A loss of extension is often the first detectable sign of effusion in the hip joint.

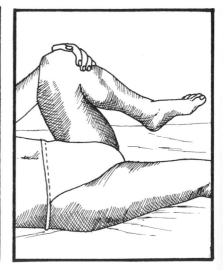

36. *Movements: Flexion* (1) The good hip is first flexed to obliterate the lumbar curve and to steady the pelvis. The patient is asked to hold the leg in this position.

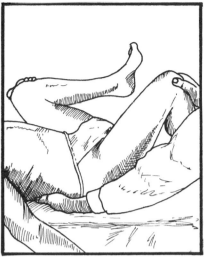

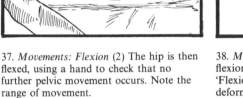

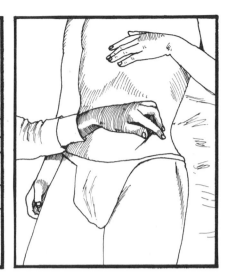

37. *Movements: Flexion* (2) The hip is then flexed, using a hand to check that no further pelvic movement occurs. Note the range of movement.
Normal range = 120°

38. *Movements: Flexion* (3) The range of flexion may be recorded in this example as 'Flexion (R) hip: 30–90°' or 'Fixed flexion deformity of 30° and hip flexes to 90°'.

39. *Movements: Abduction* (1) A false impression of hip movement may be gained if the pelvis tilts during the examination, so first place the left hand on the patient's left anterior superior iliac spine. Steady the other spine with the forearm.

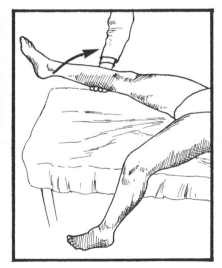

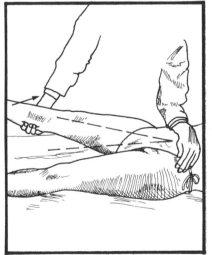

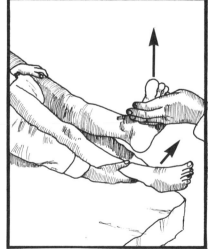

40. *Movements: Abduction* (2) An alternative way of fixing the pelvis is to flex the other leg over the edge of the couch, and check movement of the pelvis by holding the anterior superior iliac spine on the side being examined.

41. *Movements: Abduction* (3) Now having fixed the pelvis, move the leg laterally and note the range achieved.
Normal range = 40°

42. *Movements: Adduction* (1) Ideally an assistant should lift the good leg out of the way to allow the affected leg to be adducted in full extension.
Normal range = 25°

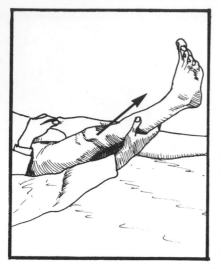

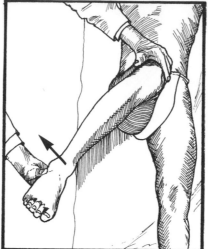

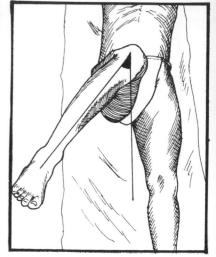

43. *Movements: Adduction* (2) If an assistant is not available cross the leg being examined over the other. This brings the leg being examined into slight flexion, but is sufficiently accurate under most circumstances. If the hip is normal, the legs should cross about mid-thigh.

44. *Movements: Rotation at 90° flexion* (1) Steady the flexed hip with one hand and move the foot laterally to produce *internal rotation of the hip.*

45. *Movements: Internal rotation at 90° flexion* (2) Measure the range of internal rotation by comparing the position of the leg and the mid-line.
Normal range = 45°
Compare the sides. Loss of internal rotation is common in most hip pathology.

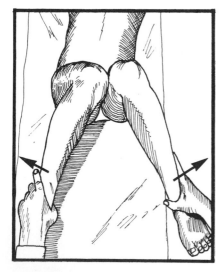

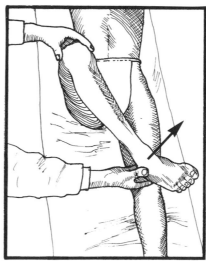

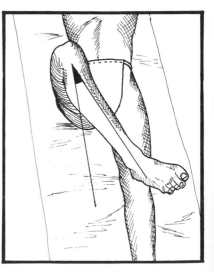

46. *Movements: Internal rotation at 90° flexion* (3) A sensitive comparison of the sides may be made by asking the patient to hold the knees together while you move both feet laterally.

47. *Movements: External rotation at 90° flexion* (1) The position of the hip is the same as for testing internal rotation, but in this case the foot is moved medially.

48. *Movements: External rotation at 90° flexion* (2) Measure external rotation in the same general way.
Normal range = 45°
External rotation becomes limited in most arthritic conditions of the hip.

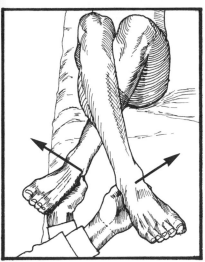

49. *Movements: External rotation at 90°
flexion* (3) Comparison between the sides
may be made by crossing one leg over the
other.

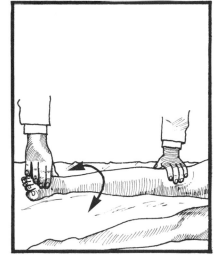

50. *Movements: Rotation in extension* (1)
For a rough comparison of the sides, roll
each leg medially and laterally, observing
any play at the knee.

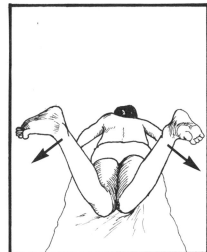

51. *Movements: Internal rotation in
extension* (2) For a more accurate
assessment, the patient should be prone,
with the knees flexed. The two sides can
easily be compared and measurements
taken.
Normal range = 35°

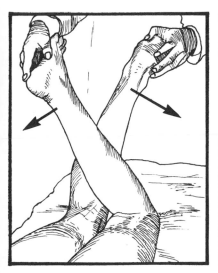

52. *Movements: External rotation in
extension* Comparison and measurement
may be made in the same way.
Normal range = 45°

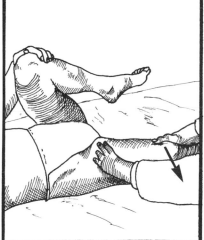

53. *Movements: Testing for hip fusion* (1)
When there is doubt regarding the solidity
of a hip fusion, it is sometimes helpful to
test for protective muscle contraction. Flex
the good hip and knee. Feel for
involuntary adductor contracture while
suddenly abducting the leg.

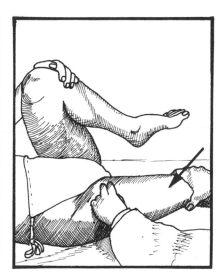

54. *Movements: Testing for hip fusion* (2)
Repeat the test, this time feeling for flexor
(ilio-psoas) contraction while making a
sudden gentle attempt to extend the hip.

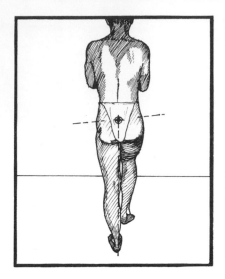

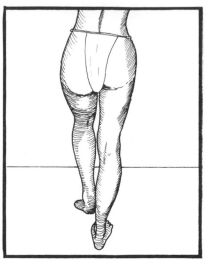

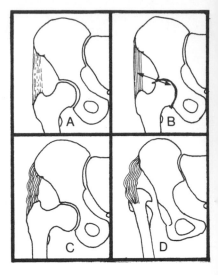

55. *Trendelenberg's test* (1) When standing on one leg, the centre of gravity (in front of S2) is brought over the weight-bearing foot by the gluteal muscles on that side tilting the pelvis. The pelvic tilt results in elevation of the buttock on the other side.

56. *Trendelenberg's test* (2) Trendelenberg's test is said to be positive when the buttock on the non-weight-bearing side fails to rise. It is associated with a typical gait (gluteal or Trendelenberg limp). If bilateral, there is a waddling gait with excessive shoulder sway.

57. *Trendelenberg's test* (3) The test is positive as a result of (A) gluteal paralysis or weakness (e.g. from polio, muscle-wasting disease), (B) gluteal inhibition (e.g. from pain arising in the hip joint), (C) from gluteal inefficiency from coxa vara or (D) CDH. Nevertheless false positives have been recorded in about 10% of patients.

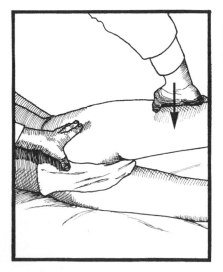

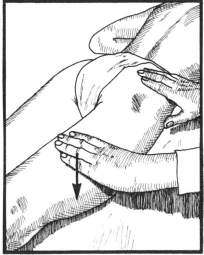

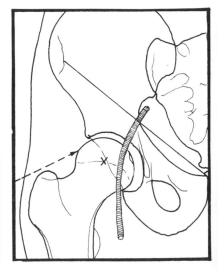

58. *Gluteal muscles:* Test the power of the abductors of the hip with the patient lying on the side, attempting to abduct the leg against resistance.

59. *Gluteal muscles:* Test the power in gluteus maximus by asking the patient to extend the hip against resistance, at the same time feeling the tone in the contracting muscle.

60. *Aspiration:* The hip may be aspirated by inserting a needle above the trochanter, allowing for femoral neck anteversion. Alternatively, a needle may be passed into the joint from in front, a little below the inguinal ligament and lateral to the femoral artery.

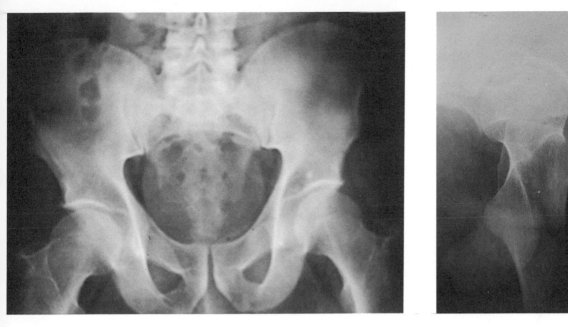

61. *Radiographs.* Normal A-P projection of the pelvis.

62. *Radiographs.* Normal lateral hip.

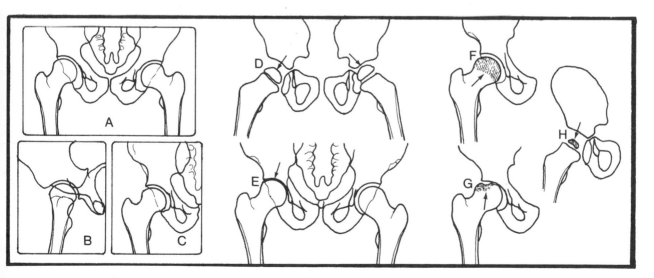

63. *Radiographs:* An A-P view showing both hips (A) is the most useful single screening film as it allows both sides to be compared. If the joint is strongly suspect, an additional lateral projection (B) and an A-P centred on the hip (C) are essential. Note first in the films any disturbance of bone texture (e.g. Paget's disease, osteoporosis, tumour). Now note the joint space (which indicates the depth of articular cartilage and interposing fluid) which may be (D) increased in Perthes' disease, synovitis and infection and (E) decreased in the later stages of infection and arthritis. Note the relative density of the femoral head which may be decreased, e.g. in rheumatoid arthritis, infection, and osteoporosis, and increased in (F) avascular necrosis (G) segmental avascular necrosis (H) Perthes' disease.

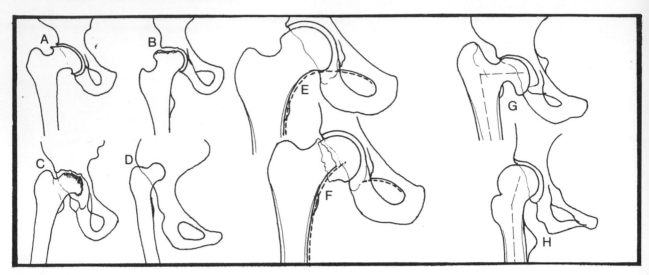

64. *Radiographs ctd:* Now note the shape of the femoral head which may for example be (A) buffer shaped after Perthe's disease, (B) flattened after avascular necrosis (total or segmental), (C) irregular or destroyed after infection, (D) atrophic in persistent congenital hip dislocation. Note Shenton's line which normally forms a smooth curve flowing from the superior pubic ramus to the femoral neck (E). Compare the sides if possible. Distortion occurs in many conditions involving the femoral neck and head, particularly fractures (F) and subluxations. Note the neck/shaft angle. This is decreased in (G) congenital coxa vara and coxa vara secondary to rickets, Paget's disease, osteo-malacia, fracture, etc. It is increased in coxa valga secondary to polio (H) and other neurological disturbances.

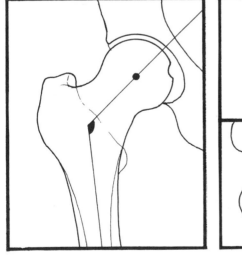

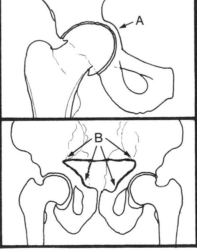

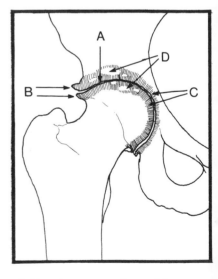

65. The neck/shaft angle may be measured from lines drawn through the shaft and along the neck into the centre of the head.
Normal angle: Males 128°
             Females 127°

66. Note any pelvic distortion such as in (A) protrusio acetabuli (often hereditary, and with associated osteo-arthritis), (B) osteo-malacia (and other diseases accompanied by bone softening, e.g. rickets, Paget's disease).

67. Note the presence of any of the changes commonly seen in osteo-arthritis, such as (A) joint space narrowing, (B) marginal osteophytes, (C) marginal sclerosis, (D) cystic changes in the head and acetabulum.

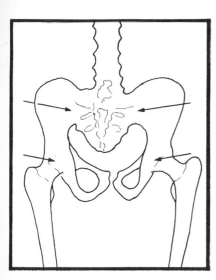

68. Complete obliteration of the hip joint (bony ankylosis) is seen in ankylosing spondylitis (where there is invariably involvement of the sacro-iliac joints). It is also seen as a late result of tuberculous and other infections, and after surgical fusion.

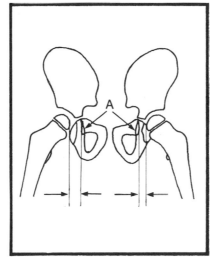

69. *Perthes' disease* (1) The earliest radiographic sign is an increase in joint space (also seen in synovitis of the hip and in infective arthritis). Minor degrees of joint widening may be detected by measuring the distance between (A) 'the tear drop' and the head on both sides.

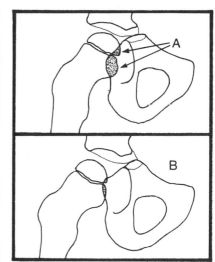

70. *Perthes' disease* (2) If the 'tear drop' (formed by the anterior acetabular floor) is not clear, note (A) the overlap shadows of the head and neck on the acetabulum, comparing one hip with the other. Alteration (B) occurs in Perthes' disease, synovitis and infection.

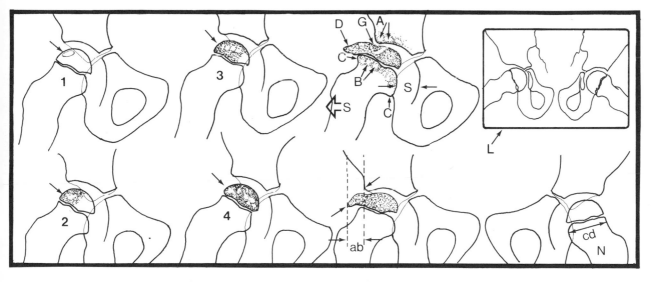

71. *Perthes' disease* (3) The severity of bone changes, when they appear, may be determined by Catterall Grading: *Grade 1:* Cyst formation occurs in the antero-lateral aspect of the capital epiphysis. Revascularisation may be completed without bone collapse, and the prognosis without treatment is good. *Grade 2:* A little more of the head is involved, and bony collapse is inevitable. *Grade 3:* Most of the head is involved. *Grade 4:* The whole head is affected. The so-called 'frog' lateral (Loewenstein) is routine in assessing these cases (L). Cystic changes may also appear in the acetabulum (A) and the metaphysis (B) which may widen (C). The femoral head may flatten and extrude laterally (D). Lateral extrusion may be expressed as a percentage of the diameter of the metaphysis on the normal (assumed) side (N): if ab/cd × 100 > 20%, then the prognosis is poor. An accurate assessment of the amount of avascular bone may be made by radionuclide bone scanning. Prognosis is mainly dependent on the mass and degree of epiphyseal involvement (assessed for example by Catterall grading). Other adverse factors placing the case in the 'head-at-risk' category include (a) presentation above the age of 4, (b) calcification seen lateral to the epiphysis or other evidence of major extrusion, (c) lateral subluxation (S), (d) a positive Gage sign (a sequestrum surrounded by a 'V' of viable epiphysis (G)).

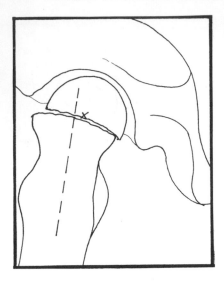

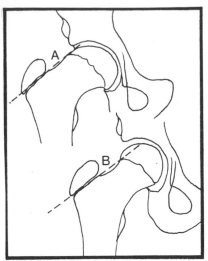

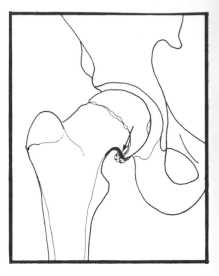

72. *Slipped femoral epiphysis* (1) The earliest changes are seen in the lateral projection. A line drawn up through the centre of the neck fails to meet the mid-point of the base of the epiphysis.

73. *Slipped femoral epiphysis* (2) Later, in the A-P view, the first sign is that a tangential line drawn on the upper femoral neck fails to strike the epiphysis (A) while in a normal well centred view such a tangent (B) includes part of the epiphysis.

74. *Slipped femoral epiphysis* (3) In the later stages, some weeks after the initial slip, there is distortion of the inferior part of the femoral neck with new bone formation (the so-called 'chronic slip').

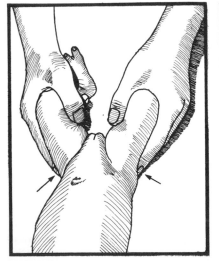

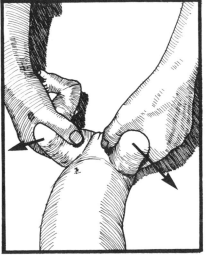

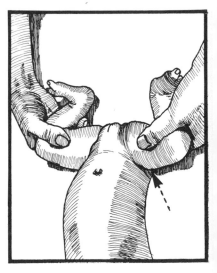

75. *Ortolani's test* (1) To be of any value the examination must be carried out on a relaxed child, preferably after feeding. Flex the knees and encircle them with the hands so that the thumbs lie along the medial sides of the thighs and the fingers over the trochanters.

76. *Ortolani's test* (2) Now flex the hips to a right angle, and starting from a position where the thumbs are touching, smoothly and gently abduct the hips.

77. *Ortolani's test* (3) If a hip is dislocated, as full abduction is approached the femoral head will be felt slipping in to the acetabulum. An audible click may accompany the displacement but in no way must this be considered an essential element of the test. Note that *restriction* of abduction may be pathological, and represent an irreducible dislocation (see also 85).

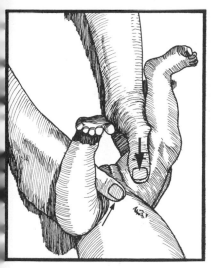

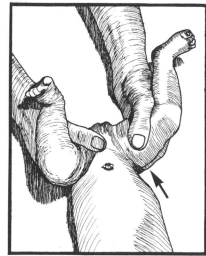

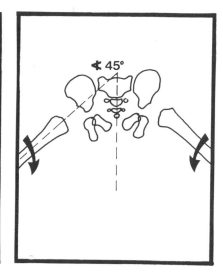

78. *Barlow's provocative test* (1) If the Ortolani test is negative the hip may nevertheless be unstable. Fix the pelvis between symphysis and sacrum with one hand. With the thumb of the other attempt to dislocate the hip by gentle but firm backward pressure. Check both sides.

79. *Barlow's test* (2) If the head of the femur is felt to sublux backwards, its reduction should be achieved by forward finger pressure or wider abduction. The movement of reduction should also be appreciated with the fingers. If either test is positive, treatment is essential.

80. *Radiographic examination:* In the neonate radiographic examination should be reserved for the doubtful case as interpretation is not completely reliable. An A-P view of the hips should be taken with the legs *in full internal rotation and abducted to not less than 45°.*

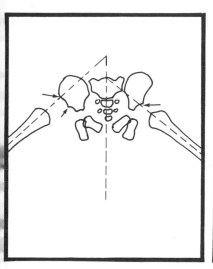

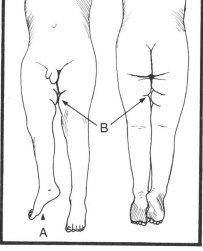

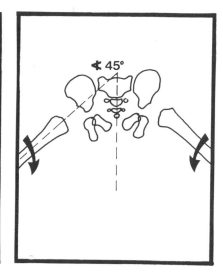

81. *Radiographic examination* (2) Draw femoral axial lines and note where their projections cut the pelvis. If the hip is in joint, the projection normally strikes the outer lip of the acetabulum. If dislocated, it will strike the ilium in the region of the anterior spine.

82. *CDH: The older child* (1) *Appearance:* (A) The affected leg in a case of unilateral congenital dislocation of the hip may appear slightly shorter, and lie in external rotation. (B) There may be asymmetry of the skin folds in the thigh although this sign is of limited reliability.

83. *CDH: The older child* (2) If both hips are involved, there is usually widening of the perineum due to the hip displacement. If the child has been walking, there will be a compensatory increase in lumbar lordosis.

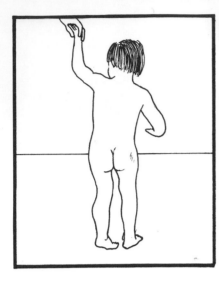

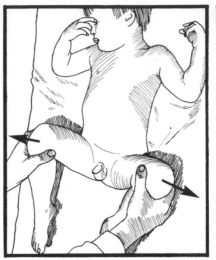

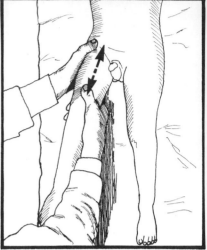

84. CDH: The older child (3)
Trendelenberg's test will be positive (see *Hip* 55) and the gait will be abnormal with excessive shoulder sway. In unilateral cases, the child will dip on the affected side: in bilateral cases the child will have a waddling gait.

85. CDH: The older child (4) Test the range of abduction from a position of 90° flexion of the hip. Abduction is restricted in CDH in this position, and of course is most obvious in the unilateral case.

86. CDH: The older child (5) Attempt to elicit telescoping in the affected limb. Steady the pelvis with one hand, and push and pull along the axis of the femur with the other. Abnormal excursion of the limb is suggestive of CDH. Always compare the sides.

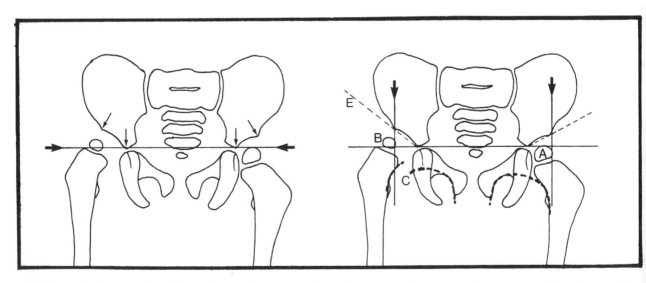

87. Radiographs: Interpretation of hip radiographs in the older child is dependent on the presence of ossification in the epiphysis of the femoral head. This normally appears between two and eight months, but is often delayed in CDH. The position of the capital epiphysis in relation to the other pelvic elements must be determined. First draw a horizontal line across the pelvis. This should touch on each side the downward pointing apex of the acetabular element of the ilium. Vertical lines should then be drawn from the lateral limit of the acetabulum. These lines divide the region of each hip in to four areas. The femoral head epiphysis should normally lie within the lower and inner quadrant (A) but in CDH the head moves upwards and outwards (as at B). (C) Shenton's line may be disturbed (see *Hip* 64). Dysplasia of the acetabulum alters its slope (E) which decreases with growth (it usually does not exceed 30° at 6 months). Additional information regarding the head, acetabulum and limbus may be obtained by contrast arthrography. The techniques and interpretation are specialised.

10 The Knee

Swelling of the knee

The knee may become swollen as a result of the accumulation within the joint cavity of excess synovial fluid, blood or pus (synovitis, haemarthrosis, pyarthrosis). Much less commonly the knee swells beyond the limits of the synovial membrane. This is seen in soft tissue injuries of the knee when haematoma and oedema may be extensive. It is also a feature of fractures, infections and tumours of the distal femur, where confusion may result either from the proximity of the lesion to the joint or its direct involvement of the cavity. Although primary tumours of the knee are rare, in malignant synovioma there is striking swelling of the joint often extending beyond the limits of the synovial cavity.

Synovitis, effusion

The synovial membrane secretes the synovial fluid of the joint; excess synovial fluid indicates some affection of the membrane. Joint injuries cause synovitis by tearing or stretching. Infections act directly by eliciting an inflammatory response which causes the synovial membrane to secrete more fluid. The membrane itself becomes thickened and abnormal in function in rheumatoid arthritis and villo-nodular synovitis, both conditions being associated with large effusions. In long standing meniscus lesions and osteo-arthrosis, the synovial membrane may not be directly involved, and consequently no effusion may be present in these conditions. Minor injuries of the knee which do not materially damage any of the main structural elements are in some cases followed by rather persistent effusions (traumatic synovitis). In spite of these exceptions, the recognition of fluid in the joint is of great importance. Effusion indicates damage to the joint, and the presence of a major lesion must always be eliminated. A tense synovitis may be aspirated to relieve discomfort.

Haemarthrosis

Blood in the knee is seen most commonly following acute injuries where there is tearing of vascular structures. The menisci are avascular, and there may be no haemarthrosis when a meniscus is torn. Bleeding into the joint will take place, however, if the meniscus has been detached at its periphery or if there is accompanying damage to other structures within the knee (e.g. the cruciate ligaments). In injuries of the medial ligament, a haematoma may track distally without involvement of the joint cavity. Nevertheless the presence of a haemarthrosis generally indicates a substantial injury to the joint. Its presence may give rise to great discomfort and make diagnosis difficult. A tense painful haemarthrosis should be aspirated.

Pyarthrosis

Infections of the knee joint are rather uncommon, and usually blood borne. Sometimes the joint is involved by direct spread from an osteitis of the femur or tibia; rarely the joint becomes infected following surgery or penetrating wounds.

In acute pyogenic infections the onset is usually rapid and the knee very painful; swelling is tense, tenderness is widespread, and movement resisted. There is pyrexia and general malaise. Pyogenic infections occurring in patients suffering from rheumatoid arthritis have often a much slower onset. Although the joint is invariably swollen, other inflammatory changes are often suppressed, especially if the patient is receiving steroids.

Tuberculous infections of the knee, now uncommon in Britain, have a slow onset spread over weeks. The knee appears small and globular with the associated profound quadriceps wasting.

In gonococcal arthritis, great pain and tenderness, often apparently out of proportion to the local swelling and other signs, are the striking features of this condition.

When pus is suspected in a joint, aspiration should always be carried out to empty it and obtain specimens for bacteriological examination. If tuberculosis is suspected, synovial biopsy to obtain specimens for culture and histology is required. All knee infections are treated by splintage and an appropriate antibiotic regime.

The extensor mechanism

Extension of the knee is produced by the quadriceps muscle acting through the quadriceps ligament, patella, patellar ligament and tibial tubercle. Weakness of extension leads to instability, repeated joint trauma and effusion. Loss of extension also leads to instability, as there is failure of the screw-home mechanism which tightens the ligaments of the joint at terminal extension.

Rapid wasting of the quadriceps is seen in all painful and inflammatory conditions of the knee. Weakness of the quadriceps is also sometimes found in lesions of the upper lumbar intervertebral discs, as a sequel to polio-myelitis, and in multiple sclerosis and other neurological disorders. Rapid quadriceps wasting is a feature of the myopathies. Difficulty in diagnosis is common when the wasting is the presenting feature of a diabetic neuropathy or secondary to femoral nerve palsy from an iliacus haematoma. Maintenance of good quadriceps tone is an essential part of the treatment of virtually all conditions affecting the knee joint.

Fractures of the patella seldom give difficulty in diagnosis provided the appropriate radiographs are taken. Rupture of the quadriceps tendon or patellar ligament result from sudden, violent contraction of the quadriceps and are seen in the middle-aged when there has been some accompanying degenerative change in the structures involved. Complete avulsion of the tibial tuberosity may also result from a sudden muscle contraction. Partial avulsion of the tuberosity in children may be the cause of Osgood-Schlatter's disease. In this condition, occurring in the 10 to 16 age group, there is recurrent pain over the tibial tuberosity which becomes tender and prominent. Pain usually ceases with closure of the epiphysis, and the management is usually conservative. Complete avulsion of the tibial tuberosity and ruptures of the quadriceps tendon and patellar ligament are treated by surgical repair.

The ligaments of the knee

The cruciate, collateral, posterior and capsular ligaments, and the menisci, form an integrated stabilising system which prevents the tibia from shifting or tilting under the femur in an abnormal fashion. The pathological movements which may occur after ligamentous injury are (a) tilting of the knee into varus or valgus, (b) shifting of the tibia directly forwards or backwards, (c) rotation of the tibia under the femur so that the medial or lateral tibial condyle subluxes forwards or backwards (see 47).

Ligament injuries are important to detect as they may account for appreciable disability in the form of incidents of giving way of the joint, recurrent effusion, lack of confidence in the knee, difficulty in undertaking strenuous or athletic activities, and sometimes trouble in using stairs or walking on uneven ground.

The diagnosis and interpretation of instability in the knee is difficult and somewhat controversial for the following reasons:

1. Several structures may be simultaneously damaged.

2. Each of the main ligamentous structures round the knee has primary and secondary supportive functions: if a ligament whose primary role in preventing a certain abnormal movement is torn, that movement may be prevented by other structures which have a secondary supporting function. Later, however, the secondary structures may stretch and give rise to increasing disability. The clinical signs in consequence may be masked initially, but become more obvious later.

3. A plethora of terms describing these instabilities makes the interpretation of the literature somewhat difficult. The present trend both in examination and management is to analyse and treat the instability; less emphasis is placed on the diagnosis of the precise anatomical disturbance. Nevertheless, the main supportive structures have certain distinctive features which should be noted.

The medial ligament and capsule

The medial ligament stretches between the femur and tibia, and has superficial and deep layers. Considerable violence (in the form of a valgus strain or blow on the side of the knee) is required to damage the medial ligament. When the forces are moderately severe, a few fibres only may be torn, usually near the upper attachment (sprain of the medial ligament). Then, when the knee is examined clinically, no instability will be demonstrated, but stretching the ligament will cause pain. Minor tears of the medial ligament may be followed eventually by calcification in the accompanying haematoma, and this may give rise to sharply localised pain at the uper attachment (Pellegrini-Stieda disease). With greater violence, the whole of the deep part of the ligament ruptures, followed in order by the superficial part, the medial capsule, the posterior ligament, the posterior cruciate ligament and sometimes finally the anterior cruciate ligament. Acute complete tears give rise to serious instability in the knee which can move or be moved in valgus. They are usually dealt with by immediate surgical repair. Partial tears do well by immobilisation for six weeks in a pipe-stem plaster. Chronic lesions may be accompanied by tibial condylar subluxation (see later) and surgical treatment may be indicated to deal with that instability. Medial ligament tears may accompany fractures of the lateral tibial table, which will require additional attention.

The lateral ligament and capsule

This ligament may be damaged by blows on the medial side of the knee, throwing it into varus. It most frequently tears at its fibular attachment. As in the case of the medial ligament, increasing violence will lead to tearing of the posterior capsular ligament and the cruciates. In addition, the common peroneal nerve may be stretched and sometimes irreversibly damaged. These injuries are usually treated by operative repair, and where applicable, exploration of the common peroneal nerve. Again, any associated fracture of the medial tibial table may require attention, and chronic lesions may be associated with tibial condylar subluxations.

The anterior cruciate ligament

Damage to the anterior cruciate ligament occurs most frequently as a sequel to tears of the medial meniscus. Many longitudinal meniscus tears produce a block to extension of the joint. Attempts to obtain full extension lead to attrition rupture of the ligament. Anterior cruciate ligament tears may also accompany severe collateral ligament injuries.

Isolated ruptures of the anterior cruciate ligament are uncommon and are not usually treated surgically unless accompanied by avulsion of bone at the anterior tibial attachment. When the tear accompanies a meniscus lesion, the meniscus is preserved if at all possible to reduce the risks of tibial subluxation and secondary osteoarthritic changes. Nevertheless, the damage may be such that excision cannot be avoided. When an acute tear is associated with damage to the collateral ligaments, a combined repair or reconstruction is usually attempted. Problems from tibial subluxation are common, particularly when anterior cruciate tears are accompanied by damage to the medial or lateral structures. When pure anterior tibial subluxation is the main source of symptoms, and these are demanding, surgical reconstruction may be indicated if simple measures such as quadriceps buildings are not successful. Methods include:

1. Using the adductor gracilis as a dynamic replacement;
2. using a tube pedicle from the ilio-tibial tract as a substitute; or
3. encouraging re-growth of ligamentous tissue by carbon fibre implants.

The posterior cruciate ligament

Posterior cruciate ligament tears are produced when in a flexed knee the tibia is forcibly pushed backwards (as for example in a car accident in which the upper part of the shin strikes the dashboard). Surgical repair is always advised if the injury is seen at the acute stage, as persisting instability and osteo-arthrosis are the usual sequelae in the untreated case.

Rotatory instability in the knee: tibial condylar subluxations

In this group of conditions, when the knee is stressed, the tibia may sublux forwards or backwards on either the medial or lateral side, giving rise to pain and a feeling of instability in the joint. The main forms are as follows:

1. *The medial tibial condyle subluxes anteriorly* (antero-medial rotatory instability): In the most severe cases, the anterior cruciate and the medial structures (medial ligament and capsule) are torn. The medial meniscus may also be damaged and contribute to the instability. In the less severe cases there is some controversy regarding which structures may be spared. Clinically, the condition should be suspected on the evidence of the anterior drawer test, and the demonstration of instability on applying a valgus stress to the joint.

2. *The lateral tibial condyle subluxes anteriorly* (antero-lateral rotatory instability): In the more severe cases the anterior cruciate ligament and lateral structures are torn, and there may be an associated lesion of the anterior horn of the lateral meniscus. It may be diagnosed from the results of the anterior drawer test and by demonstrating instability on applying a varus stress to the knee, although a number of specific tests may afford additional confirmation.

3. *The lateral tibial condyle subluxes posteriorly* (postero-lateral rotatory instability): This may follow rupture of the lateral and posterior cruciate ligaments, and be recognised by the presence of instability in the knee on applying varus stress associated with an abnormal posterior drawer test.

4. *Combinations of these lesions* (particularly 1 & 2, and 2 & 3) may be found, especially where there is major ligamentous disruption of the knee.

Where symptoms are demanding, and when a firm diagnosis has been established, the stability of the joint may be restored by an appropriate ligamentous reattachment or reinforcement procedure.

Lesions of the menisci

Congenital discoid meniscus

This abnormality, most frequently involving the lateral meniscus, commonly gives rise to presenting symptoms in childhood. The meniscus has not its usual semilunar form, but is rather more D-shaped, with its central edge extending in towards the tibial spines. It may produce a very pronounced clicking from the lateral compartment, a block to extension of the joint, and other derangement signs. It is treated by excision.

Meniscus tears in the young adult

The commonest cause is a sporting injury when a twisting strain is applied to the flexed, weight-bearing leg. The entrapped meniscus commonly splits longitudinally, and its free edge may displace inwards towards the centre of the joint (bucket-handle tear). This prevents full extension (locking) and if an attempt is made to straighten the knee, a painful elastic resistance is felt (springy block to full extension). In the case of the medial meniscus, prolonged loss of full extension may lead to stretching and eventual rupture of the anterior cruciate ligament. Lateral meniscus tears are often associated with cysts of the meniscus which restrict its mobility. Meniscus tears are treated by excision of the meniscus, but in the case of bucket-handle tears, removal of the central portion only may decrease the risks of late secondary osteo-arthritis.

Degenerative meniscus lesions in the middle-aged

Loss of elasticity in the menisci through degenerative changes associated with the ageing process may give rise to horizontal cleavage tears within the substance of the meniscus; these tears may not be associated with any remembered incident, and sharply localised tenderness in the joint line is a common feature. In an appreciable number of cases symptoms may resolve without surgery, although excision may sometimes be required.

Cysts of the menisci

Ganglion-like cysts occur in both menisci, but are much more common in the lateral. There is often a history of a blow on the side of the knee over the meniscus. They are tender, and as they restrict the mobility of the menisci, they render them more susceptible to tears. They are treated by excision, and in most cases, simultaneous meniscectomy. Medial meniscus cysts must be carefully distinguished from ganglions arising from the pes anserinus (the insertion of sartorius, gracilis and semitendinosus).

Recurrent dislocation of the patella

A traumatic incident usually produces the first lateral dislocation of the patella which is accompanied by pain and deformity. The patella may reduce spontaneously or require manipulative reduction. Subsequently the patella may dislocate with progressive ease, and in long standing cases may remain permanently displaced on the lateral side of the joint. The first incident characteristically occurs in adolescence, and is much commoner in girls than in boys. It is often associated with knock knees, a mild degree of genu recurvatum and a highly placed patella, an underdeveloped lateral femoral condyle and sometimes an abnormal quadriceps attachment to femur and patella. In the young, before the tibial epiphysis has closed, recurrent dislocation may be treated by using the distal part of the tendon of semitendinosus to stabilise the patella (Galeazzi repair). When the epiphysis is closed, the tuberosity may be transposed medially and distally, altering the line of pull of the quadriceps and thereby stabilising the patella (Hauser operation).

Chondromalacia patellae

In this condition, most common in girls and young women, the articular cartilage of the patella becomes soft and spongy, giving rise to aching pain in the front of the knee. It may follow recurrent dislocation of the patella, and may progress to retro-patellar osteo-arthrosis. Early cases are treated by a period of immobilisation in plaster, and more severe cases by paring the articular surface of the patella at operation. Where the changes are very advanced, patellectomy may be required to avoid future osteo-arthrosis.

Osteochondritis dissecans

This occurs most frequently in males in the second decade of life, and most commonly involves the medial femoral condyle. Possibly as a result of impingement against the tibial spines or the cruciate ligaments, a segment of bone undergoes avascular necrosis, and a line of demarcation becomes established between this area and the underlying healthy bone. Complete separation may occur so that a loose body is formed. The symptoms are initially of aching pain and recurring effusion, with perhaps locking of the joint if a loose body is present. The treatment is usually surgical. Before separation, attempts may be made to revascularise the interface by drilling through this area into the underlying healthy bone. After separation, attempts are sometimes made to replace the loose fragment with fine steel pins. In all cases, the damaging effects of a loose body must be prevented.

Fat pad injuries

The infrapatellar fat pads may become tender and swollen and give rise to pain on extension of the knee, especially if they are nipped between the articulating surfaces of femur and tibia. This may occur as a complication of osteo-arthrosis, but is seen more frequently in young women when the fat pads swell in association with premenstrual fluid retention. Excision of the pads may be required to relieve the symptoms.

Loose bodies

Loose bodies are seen most frequently as a sequel to osteo-arthrosis or osteochondritis dissecans. Much less commonly, numerous loose bodies are formed by an abnormal synovial membrane in the condition of synovial chondromatosis. Loose bodies are treated by excision, but synovectomy may be required in synovial chondromatosis if massive recurrence is to be avoided.

Affections of the articular surfaces

Osteo-arthrosis (osteo-arthritis)

The stresses of weight-bearing mainly involve the medial compartment of the knee, and it is in this area that primary osteo-arthrosis usually first occurs. This is an exceedingly common condition, arising without any obvious previous pathology in the joint. Overweight, the degenerative changes accompanying old age, and overwork are common factors. Secondary osteo-arthrosis may follow ligament and meniscus injuries, recurrent dislocation of the patella, osteochondritis dissecans, joint infections and other previous pathology. It is seen in association with knock knee and bow leg deformities which throw additional mechanical stresses on the joint.

In osteo-arthrosis, the articular cartilage undergoes progressive change, flaking off into the joint and thereby producing the narrowing that is a striking feature of radiographs of this condition. The subarticular bone may become eburnated, and often small marginal osteophytes and cysts are formed. Exposure of bone and free nerve endings gives rise to pain and crepitations on movement. Distortion of the joint surfaces is one cause of progressive loss of movement and fixed flexion deformities. Treatment is generally conservative, by quadriceps exercises, short wave diathermy, analgesics and weight reduction. Surgery may be considered in severe cases. The procedures available include osteotomy (especially in cases of genu varum and valgum), arthrodesis, and joint replacement.

Rheumatoid arthritis

Characteristically the knee is warm to touch, there is effusion, limitation of movements, muscle wasting, synovial thickening, tenderness and pain. Fixed flexion, varus and valgus deformities are quite common. Generally several joints are involved, although the mono-articular form is occasionally seen. Active cases are often treated by synovectomy in an attempt to avoid or delay the progress of the condition. An acute flare up of symptoms may be treated by temporary splintage. Arthrodesis, osteotomy or knee replacement procedures are carried out in well selected cases.

Reiter's syndrome

This usually presents as a chronic effusion accompanied by discomfort in the joint. It is often bilateral, with an associated conjunctivitis. There is often a history of urethritis or colitis.

Ankylosing spondylitis

The first symptoms of ankylosing spondylitis are generally in the spine, but occasionally it presents at the periphery with swelling and discomfort in the knee joint. Stiffness of the spine and radiographic changes in the sacro-iliac joints are nevertheless almost invariably present.

Disturbances of alignment

Genu varum (bow leg)

This commonly occurs as a growth abnormality of early childhood, and usually resolves spontaneously. Rarely genu varum is caused by a growth disturbance involving both the tibial epiphysis and proximal tibial shaft (tibia vara) and treatment by osteotomy may be required. In adults this deformity most frequently results from osteo-arthrosis, where there is narrowing of the medial joint compartment. It also occurs in Paget's disease, rheumatoid arthritis and rickets.

Genu valgum (knock knee)

This is seen most often in young children where it is usually associated with flat foot. Nearly all cases resolve spontaneously by the age of six. It is also seen in the plump adolescent girl, and may be a contributory factor in recurrent dislocation of the patella. In adults it most frequently occurs as a result of the bone softening and ligamentous stretching accompanying rheumatoid arthritis. It occurs after uncorrected fractures of the lateral tibial table with depression, and as a sequel to a number of paralytic neurological disorders where there is ligament stretching and altered epiphyseal growth. Selected cases may be treated by corrective osteotomy.

Genu recurvatum

Hyperextension at the knee is seen after ruptures of the anterior cruciate ligament and in girls where the growth of the upper tibial epiphysis may be retarded from the wearing of high heeled shoes in early adolescence. In the latter case, there is a corresponding elevation of the patella contributing to a tendency to recurrent dislocation. More rarely, the deformity is seen in congenital joint laxity, poliomyelitis and Charcot's disease.

Bursitis

Cystic swelling occurring in the popliteal region in both sexes is usually referred to as enlargement of the semimembranosus bursa. In fact several of the bursae known to the anatomist may be involved — singly or together — and the swelling sometimes communicates with the knee joint itself. If there is any doubt about the diagnosis, or if the swelling is persistent and producing symptoms, excision is advised.

Fluctuant bursal swellings may also occur over the patella (prepatellar bursitis) or the patellar ligament (infrapatellar bursitis). If the swelling is bulky or tense it is aspirated; recurrent swellings, if troublesome, are excised.

How to diagnose a knee complaint

1. Note the patient's age and sex, bearing in mind the following important distribution of the common knee conditions.

Age group	Males	Females
0–12	Discoid lateral meniscus	Discoid lateral meniscus
12–18	Osteochondritis dissecans	First incidents of recurrent dislocation of the patella
	Osgood–Schlatter's disease	Osgood–Schlatter's disease
18–30	Longitudinal meniscus tears	Recurrent dislocation of the patella
		Chondromalacia patellae
		Fat pad injury
30–50	Rheumatoid arthritis	Rheumatoid arthritis
40–55	Degenerative meniscus lesions	Degenerative meniscus lesions
45+	Osteo-arthrosis	Osteo-arthrosis

Infections are comparatively uncommon and occur in both sexes in all age groups.

Reiter's syndrome occurs in adults of both sexes; ankylosing spondylitis nearly always occurs in male adults. Both are comparatively rare.

Ligamentous and extensor apparatus injuries occur in both sexes, but are rare in children.

2. Find out if the knee swells. An effusion indicates the presence of pathology which must be determined. (Note however that the absence of effusion does not necessarily eliminate significant pathology.)

3. Try to establish whether there is a mechanical problem (internal derangement) accounting for the patient's symptoms. Do this by

a. *obtaining a convincing history of an initiating injury.* Note the degree of violence, and its direction. The initial incapacity is important. For example, a footballer is unlikely to be able to finish a game with a freshly torn meniscus. Note whether there was bruising or swelling after the injury, and whether the patient was able to weight-bear.

b. *asking if the knee 'gives way'.* 'Giving way' of the knee on going down stairs or jumping from a height follows cruciate ligament tears, loss of full extension in the knee, and quadriceps wasting. 'Giving way' on twisting movements or walking on uneven ground follows many meniscus injuries.

c. *asking if the knee 'locks'.* Patients often confuse stiffness and true locking. Ask the patient to show the position the knee is in if it locks. Remember that the knee never locks in full extension. Locking due to a torn meniscus generally allows the joint to be flexed fully or nearly fully, but the last 10 to 40° of extension are impossible. Attempts to obtain full extension are accompanied by pain. Ask what produces any locking. With long standing meniscus lesions a slight rotational force, such as the foot catching on the edge of a carpet, may be quite sufficient. In chronic lesions weight-bearing is not an essential factor, locking not infrequently occuring during sleep. If the knee is not locked at the time of the patient's attendance, ask how it became free: unlocking with a click is suggestive of a meniscus lesion. Locking from a loose body may occur at varying positions of flexion. Locking from a dislocating patella may be noted to be accompanied by deformity.

d. *asking about pain.* Find out the circumstances in which it is present and ask the patient if he can localise it by pointing with one finger to the site.

In a high proportion of cases the likely diagnosis will have been established by this stage, requiring only confirmation by clinical examination.

Additional investigations

Occasionally a firm diagnosis cannot be made on the basis of the history and clinical examination alone. The following additional investigations are often helpful.

Suspected internal derangement

a. *Provocative exercises.* These are carried out under the supervision of a trained physiotherapist. They aim to throw considerable stress on the menisci by applying torsional stresses to the weight-bearing knee. If the meniscus has been damaged, the exercises are likely to be followed by localised pain, swelling and sometimes even locking—so that any doubtful meniscus lesion is likely to declare itself.

b. *Examination under anaesthesia.* If pain prevents full examination (e.g. by preventing flexion) anaesthesia may be helpful.

c. Arthroscopy and/or arthrography may give much useful information, and in conjunction with the clinical examination will allow a firm, accurate diagnosis to be made in the majority of cases.

d. Exploration may still be required in the occasional difficult case.

Suspected acute infections

a. Aspiration and culture of the synovial fluid.
b. Blood culture.
c. Full blood count including differential white count, and estimation of the sedimentation rate.

Suspected tuberculosis of the knee

a. Chest radiograph.
b. Synovial biopsy, with specimens of synovial membrane being sent for both histological and bacteriological examination. At the same time, synovial fluid specimens are also sent for bacteriology.
c. Mantoux test.

Suspected rheumatoid arthritis

a. Examination of other joints.
b. Rose-Waaler and Latex fixation tests.
c. Full blood count and estimation of the sedimentation rate.
d. Serum uric acid estimation.

Further investigation of poor mineralisation, bone erosions, etc.

a. Estimation of serum calcium, phosphate and alkaline phosphatase.
b. Rose-Waaler and Latex fixation tests.
c. Serum uric acid estimation.
d. Full blood count and differential count.
e. Skeletal survey and chest radiograph.
f. Bone biopsy.

Further investigation of chronic effusion, aspirate negative

a. Tests as for suspected rheumatoid arthritis.
b. Brucellosis agglutination tests.
c. Radiography of the chest and sacro-iliac joints.
d. Exploration and synovial biopsy.

Further investigation of severe undiagnosed pain

a. Radiography of the chest, pelvis and hips.
b. Exploration.

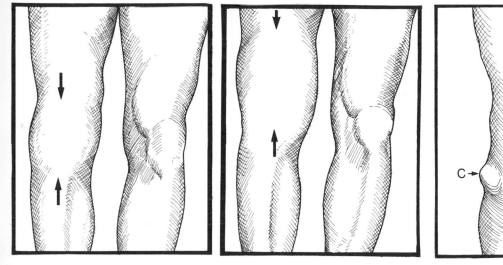

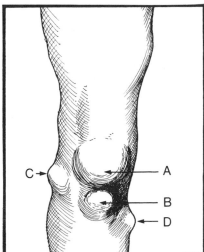

1. *Swelling:* (1) Note the presence of swelling confined to the limits of the synovial cavity and suprapatellar pouch — suggesting effusion, haemarthrosis, pyarthrosis or a space occupying lesion in the joint.

2. *Swelling:* (2) Note if the swelling extends beyond the limits of the joint cavity, suggesting infection (of the joint, femur or tibia), tumour or major injury.

3. *Lumps:* Note presence of localised swellings, e.g. (A) pre-patellar bursitis, (B) infra-patellar bursitis, (C) meniscus cyst (in joint line), (D) diaphyseal aclasis (exostosis, often multiple and sometimes familial).

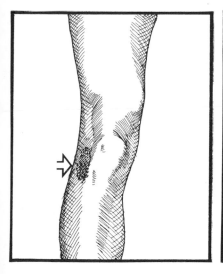

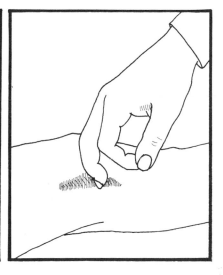

4. *Discolouration:* Note bruising, suggesting trauma to the superficial tissues, or ligament injuries (bruising is not usually seen in meniscus injuries). Note any redness suggesting inflammation.

5. *Skin marks:* Note (A) scars of previous injury or surgery — the relevant history *must* be obtained. (B) Sinus scars indicate old infection. (C) Note that arthritis and psoriasis are often associated.

6. *Temperature:* (1) Note any increased local heat and its extent, suggesting in particular rheumatoid arthritis or infection. Always compare the two sides.

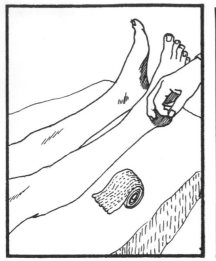

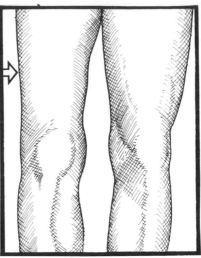

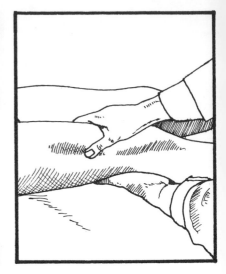

7. *Temperature:* (2) A warm knee and cold foot suggest a popliteal artery block. Always make allowance for any warm bandage the patient may have been wearing just prior to the examination.

8. *The Quadriceps:* (1) Inspect the relaxed quadriceps muscle. Slight wasting and loss of bulk are normally apparent on careful inspection.

9. *The Quadriceps:* (2) Examine the contracted quadriceps. Place a hand behind the knee and ask the patient to press the leg against the hand. Feel the muscle tone with the free hand.

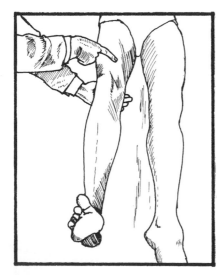

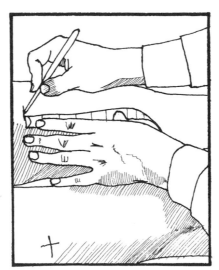

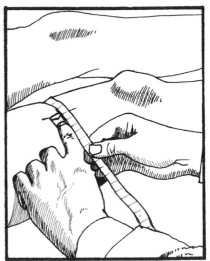

10. *The Quadriceps:* (3) Repeat the last test, this time asking the patient to dorsiflex the inverted foot. This demonstrates the important vastus medialis portion of the quadriceps, which is particularly involved in recurrent dislocation of the patella.

11. *The Quadriceps:* (4) Substantial wasting, especially in the fat leg, may be confirmed by measurement, assuming the other limb is normal. This may be valuable in medico-legal cases. Begin by marking a point 18 cm above the joint line. Do this on both legs.

12. *The Quadriceps* (5) Compare the circumference of the legs at the marked levels. Wasting of the quadriceps occurs most frequently as the result of disuse, generally from a painful or unstable lesion of the knee, or from infection or rheumatoid arthritis.

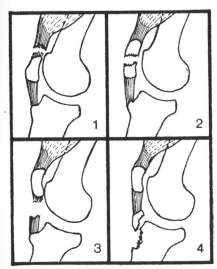

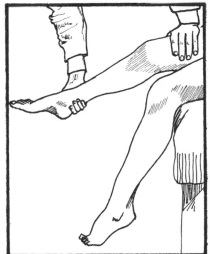

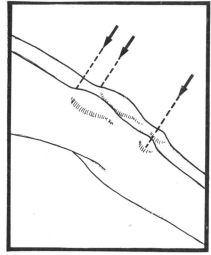

13. *Extensor Apparatus:* (1) Loss of active extension of the knee (excluding paralytic conditions) follows (1) rupture of the quadriceps tendon, (2) many patellar fractures, (3) rupture of the patellar ligament, (4) avulsion of the tibial tubercle.

14. *Extensor Apparatus:* (2) Ask the patient to straighten the leg while supporting the ankle with one hand. Feel for quadriceps contraction, and look for active extension of the limb.

15. *Extension Apparatus:* (3) Note the position of the patella. If the upper border is high suspect lesions 2, 3, or 4.

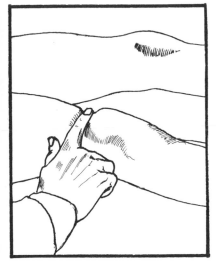

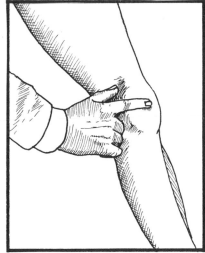

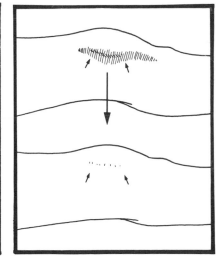

16. *Extensor Apparatus:* (4) If the patella is normally placed, lay a finger along its upper border. Loss of normal soft tissue resistance is suggestive of a rupture of the quadriceps tendon (1).

17. *Extensor Apparatus:* (5) Look for gaps and tenderness at the other levels to help differentiate between lesions, 2, 3, and 4. Radiographs of the knee are essential.

18. *Effusion:* (1) Small effusions are detected most easily by inspection. The first signs are bulging at the sides of the patellar ligament and obliteration of the hollows at the medial and lateral edges of the patella.

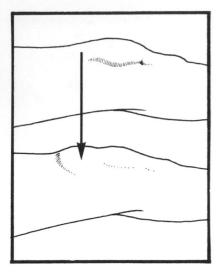

19. *Effusion:* (2) With greater effusion into the knee the suprapatellar pouch becomes distended. Effusion indicates synovial irritation from trauma or inflammation.

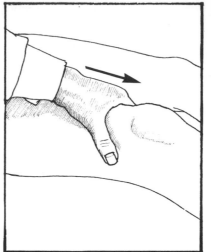

20. *Effusion:* (3) *Patellar tap:* Squeeze any excess fluid out of the suprapatellar pouch with the index and thumb, slid firmly distally from a point about 15 cm above the knee to the level of the upper border of the patella.

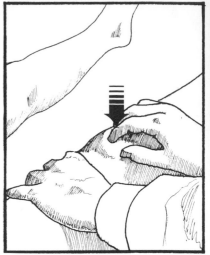

21. *Effusion:* (4) *Patellar tap:* Place the tips of the thumb and three fingers of the free hand squarely on the patella, and jerk it quickly downwards. A click indicates the presence of effusion. If, however, the effusion is slight or tense, the tap test will be negative.

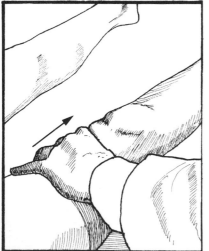

22. *Effusion:* (5) *Fluid displacement test:* Small effusions may be detected by this manoeuvre. Evacuate the suprapatellar pouch as before in the patellar tap test.

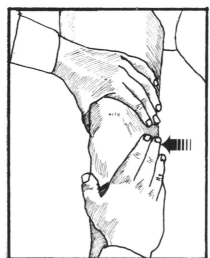

23. *Effusion:* (6) *Fluid displacement test:* Stroke the medial side of the joint to displace any excess fluid in the main joint cavity to the lateral side of the joint.

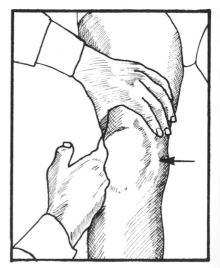

24. *Effusion:* (7) *Fluid displacement:* Now stroke the lateral side of the joint while watching closely the medial. Any excess fluid present will be seen to move across the joint and distend the medial side. This test will be negative if the effusion is gross and tense.

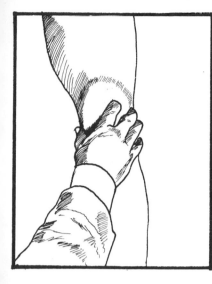

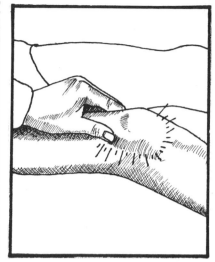

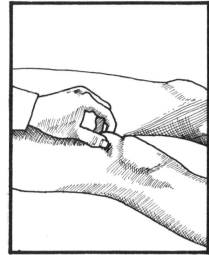

25. *Haemarthrosis:* A haemarthrosis is usually obvious within half an hour of injury, and gives a doughy feel in the suprapatellar region. A tense haemarthrosis should be aspirated to relieve pain and permit a more thorough examination of other structures.

26. *Pyarthrosis:* Tenderness in pyarthrosis is usually widespread. There is generally a severe systemic upset, and quadricepts wasting. If pyarthrosis is suspected, the knee should always be aspirated.

27. *Synovial Membrane:* Pick up the skin and the relaxed quadriceps tendon to assess the thickness of the synovial membrane in the suprapatellar pouch. The synovial membrane is thickened in inflammatory conditions, e.g. rheumatoid arthritis, and in villo-nodular synovitis.

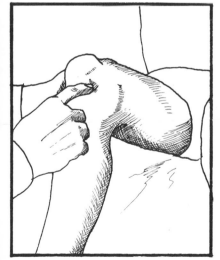

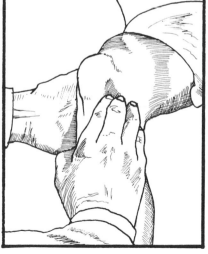

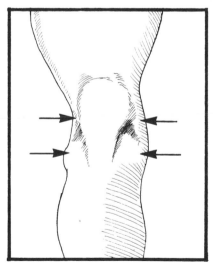

28. *Tenderness:* (1) It is a first essential to identify the joint line quite clearly. First flex the knee, and look for the hollows at the sides of the patellar ligament; these lie over the joint line.

29. *Tenderness:* (2) *Joint line structures:* Begin by palpating carefully from before back along the joint line on each side. Localised tenderness here is commonest in meniscus, collateral ligament and fat pad injuries.

30. *Tenderness:* (4) *Collateral ligaments:* Now systematically examine the upper and lower attachments of the collateral ligaments. Associated bruising and oedema is a feature of acute injuries.

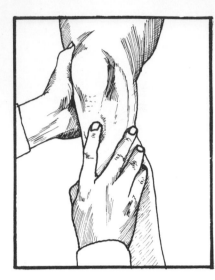

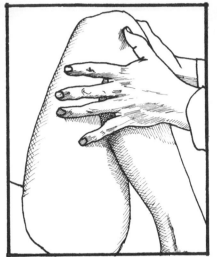

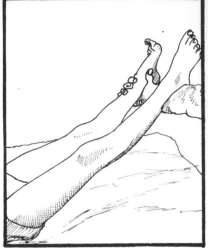

31. *Tenderness:* (4) *Tibial tubercle:* In children and adolescents, tenderness is found over the tibial tubercle (which may be prominent) in Osgood-Schlatter's disease and after acute avulsion injuries of the patellar ligament and its tibial attachment.

32. *Tenderness:* (5) *Femoral condyles:* In suspected osteo-chondritis dissecans, flex the knee fully and look for tenderness over the femoral condyles. Osteochondritis dissecans most frequently involves the medial femoral condyle, and particular attention should therefore be paid to that side.

33. *Movements:* (1) *Extension:* First make sure that the knee can be fully extended. If in doubt, lift both legs and sight along the good and affected leg. Full extension is recorded as 0°. Loss of full extension may be recorded as 'The knee lacks X° of extension'.

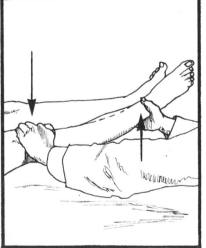

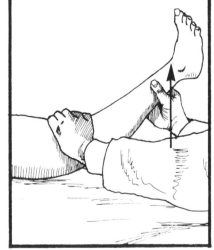

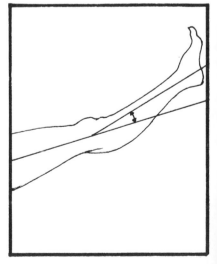

34. *Movements:* (2) *Extension:* Try to obtain full extension if this is not present. A springy block to full extension is very suggestive of a bucket handle meniscus tear. A rigid block to full extension is common in arthritic conditions (fixed flexion deformity).

35. *Movements:* (3) *Hyperextension* (genu recurvatum): This is present if the knee extends beyond the point when the tibia and femur are in line. Attempt to demonstrate this by lifting the leg while at the same time pressing back on the patella.

36. *Movements:* (4) *Hyperextension,* if present, is recorded as 'X° hyperextension'. It is seen most often in girls, often being associated with a high patella, chondromalacia patellae, recurrent patellar dislocation, and sometimes tears of the anterior cruciate, medial ligament, or medial meniscus.

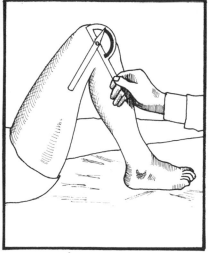

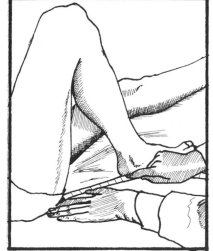

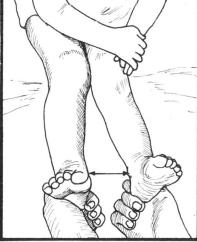

37. *Movements:* (5) *Flexion* (1) Measure in degrees from the zero position of normal full extension. Flexion of 135° and over is regarded as normal; but compare the sides. There are many causes of loss of flexion, the commonest of which are effusion and arthritic conditions.

38. *Movements:* (6) *Flexion* (2) Alternatively, measure the heel to buttock distance with the leg fully flexed. This can be a very accurate way of detecting small alterations in the range (1 cm = 1.5° approx.) and is useful for checking daily or weekly progress.

39. *Movements:* (7) *Recording:* The range of movements in the examples would be recorded as follows:
(A) *0–135°* (*normal range*)
(B) 5° hyperextension–140° flexion
(C) 10°–60°

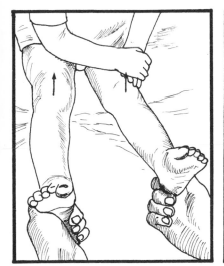

40. *Genu Valgum* (*knock knee*) *in children:* (1) Note whether unilateral, or as is usual, bilateral. The severity of the deformity is recorded by measuring the inter-malleolar gap. Grasp the child by the ankles, and rotate the legs until the patellae are vertical.

41. *Genu Valgum in children:* (2) Now bring the legs together to touch *lightly* at the knees, and measure the gap between the malleoli. Serial measurements, often every six months, are used to check progress. Note that with growth, a static measurement is an angular improvement.

42. *Genue Valgum in adults:* (1) In adults the deformity is often secondary to osteo-arthritis or rheumatoid arthritis, and it is also common in teenage girls. It is best measured by X-ray, and the films should be taken with the patient taking all his weight on the affected side.

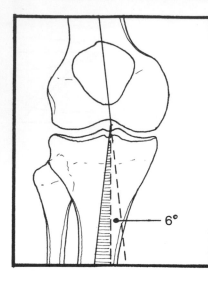

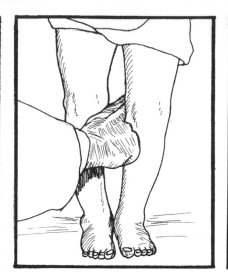

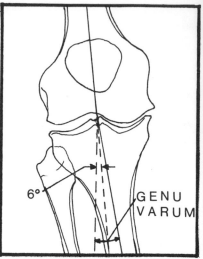

43. *Genu Valgum in adults:* (2) The degree of valgus may be roughly assessed by measuring the angle formed by the tibial and femoral shafts. Allow for the 'normal' angle which is approximately 6° in the adult. The shaded area represents genu valgum.

44. *Genu Varum* (*Bow Leg*): (1) Measure the distance between the knees, using the fingers as a gauge. Ideally the patient should be weight-bearing, and it is essential that both patellae should be facing forwards to counter any effect of hip rotation.

45. *Genu Varum:* (2) An assessment of the deformity may also be carried out radiographically, as in Genu Valgum. The deformity is seen most commonly in osteo-arthritis, rheumatoid arthritis and Paget's disease.

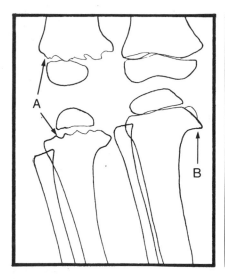

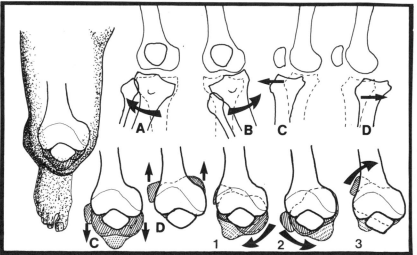

46. *Genu Varum:* (3) In children, radiography may be helpful. In (A) rickets note the wide and irregular epiphyseal plates. In (B) tibia vara note the sharply downturned medial metaphyseal border. Note that radiological varus is *normal* till a child is 18 months old.

47. *Instability in the knee:* The following potential deformities may be looked for: (A) *Valgus* (when the medial ligament is torn: severe when the posterior cruciate is also damaged). (B) *Varus* (when the lateral ligament is torn: severe when the posterior cruciate is also torn). (C) *Anterior displacement of the tibia* (anterior cruciate tears: worse if medial and/or lateral structures torn). (D) *Posterior displacement of the tibia* (posterior cruciate ligament tears). (E) *Rotatory*, with the following sub-divisions: (1) *The medial tibial condyle subluxes anteriorly* (antero-medial instability): (occurs mainly with tears of the anterior cruciate and medial structures together). (2) *The lateral condyle subluxes anteriorly* (antero-lateral instability): (mainly anterior cruciate with the lateral structures). (3) *The lateral tibial condyle subluxes posteriorly* (postero-lateral instability): (mainly tears of the posterior cruciate and lateral structures). (4) *Combinations of 1 & 2 or 2 & 3.* (Stippled drawing shows aspect of bottom 5 diagrams.)

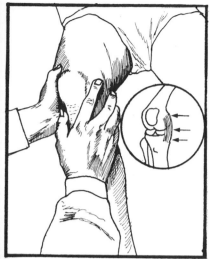

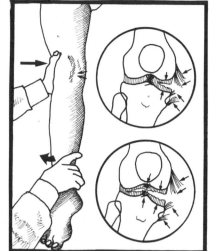

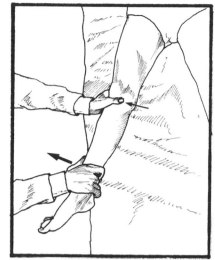

48. *Valgus stress instability:* (1) Begin by examining the medial side of the joint, and the medial ligament in particular. Tenderness in injuries of the medial ligament is commonest at the upper (femoral) attachment and in the medial joint line. Bruising may be present after recent trauma, but haemarthrosis may be absent.

49. *Valgus stress instability:* (2) Extend the knee fully. Use one hand as a fulcrum, and with the other attempt to abduct the leg. Look for the joint opening up, and the leg going in to valgus. Moderate valgus is suggestive of a major medial and posterior ligament rupture. Severe valgus indicates additional cruciate (particularly posterior cruciate) rupture.

50. *Valgus stress instability:* (3) If in doubt, use the heel of the hand as a fulcrum, and use the thumb or index, placed in the joint line, to detect any opening up of the joint as it is stressed. If there is still some uncertainty, compare the two sides.

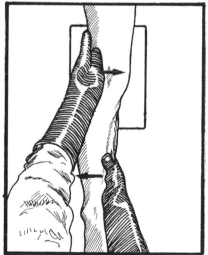

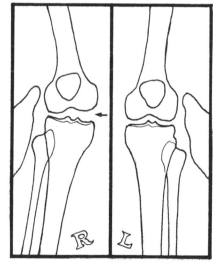

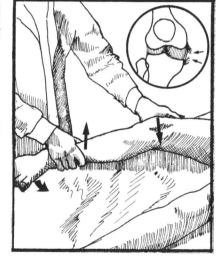

51. *Valgus stress instability:* (4) *Stress films:* If there is still some doubt, then radiographs of both knees should be taken while applying a valgus stress to each joint.

52. *Valgus stress instability:* (5) *Stress films:* The films of both sides are then compared. Any instability should be obvious.

53. *Valgus stress instability:* (6) If no instability has been demonstrated with the knee fully extended, repeat the tests with the knee flexed to 30° and the foot internally rotated. Some opening up of the joint is normal, and it is essential to compare sides. Demonstration of an abnormal amount of valgus suggests less extensive involvement of the medial structures.

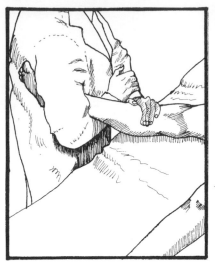

54. *Valgus stress instability:* (7) If the knee is very tender, and will not permit the pressure of a hand as a fulcrum, attempt to stress the ligament with this cross-over arm grip.

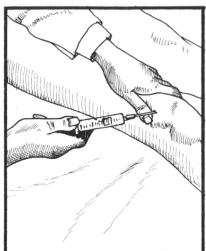

55. *Valgus stress instability:* (8) If a haemarthrosis is present (and this is not always the case) preliminary aspiration of the joint may make a useful examination possible.

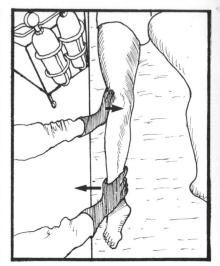

56. *Valgus stress instability:* (9) If the knee remains too painful to permit examination, the joint should be fully tested under anaesthesia; there should be provision to carry on with a surgical repair should major instability be demonstrated.

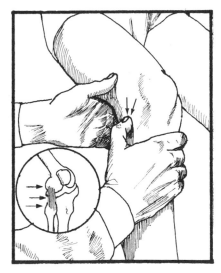

57. *Varus stress instability:* (1) Begin by examining the lateral side of the joint. Tenderness is most common over the head of the fibula or in the lateral joint line in acute injuries of the lateral joint complex (lateral ligament and capsùle).

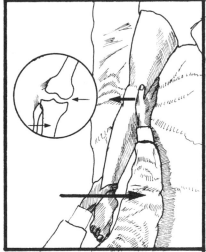

58. *Varus stress instability:* (2) Attempt to produce a varus deformity by placing one hand on the medial side of the joint and forcing the ankle medially. Carry out the test as in the case of valgus stress instability first in full extension and then in 30° flexion, and compare one side with the other.

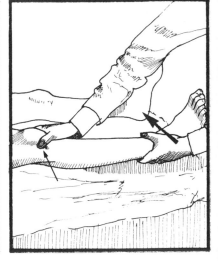

59. *Varus stress instability:* (3) Again, for a more sensitive assessment of 'give', the thumb can be placed in the joint line. If there is varus instability in extension as well as flexion, it suggests tearing of the posterior cruciate ligament as well as the lateral ligament complex.

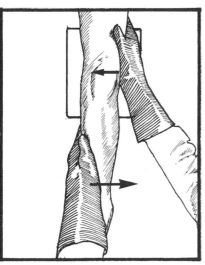

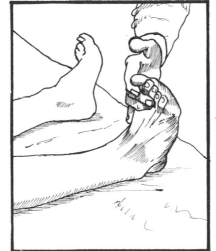

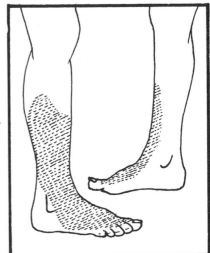

60. *Varus stress instability:* (4) As in the case of valgus stress instability, stress films may be taken, and if examination is not possible even after aspiration, arrange to examine the knee under general anaesthesia.

61. *Varus stress instability:* (5) Always check that the patient is able to dorsiflex the foot, to ensure that the motor fibres in the common peroneal nerve (lateral popliteal) have escaped damage.

62. *Varus stress instability:* (6) In addition, test for sensory disturbance in the distribution of the common peroneal nerve.

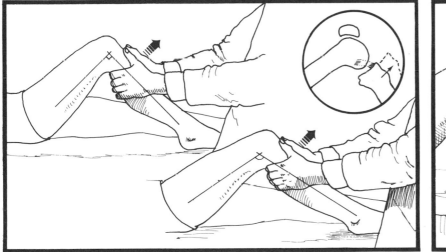

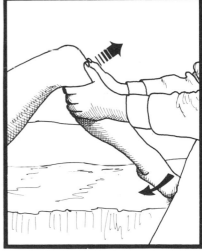

63. *The anterior drawer test:* (1) Flex the knee to 90°, see that the foot is pointing straight forwards, and steady it by sitting close to it. Grasp the leg firmly with the thumbs on the tibial tubercle. Check that the hamstrings are relaxed, and jerk the leg towards you. Repeat with the knee flexed to 70°, and compare the sides. Note: significant dispacement (i.e. the affected side more than the other) confirms instability of the type in which the tibia may move anteriorly from under the femur. When the displacement is marked (say 1.5 cm or more), then the anterior cruciate is almost certainly torn, and there is a strong possibility of associated damage to the medial complex (medial ligament and medial capsule) and even the lateral complex as well. If the displacement is less marked and one tibial condyle moves further forward than the other, then the diagnosis is less clear: it may suggest an isolated anterior cruciate ligament tear or a tibial condylar subluxation (rotatory instability).

64. *The anterior drawer test:* (2) Now turn the foot in to 15° of external rotation and repeat the test. Increased anterior excursion of the medial tibial condyle suggests rotatory instability of the type in which the medial tibial condyle subluxes forwards (antero-medial rotatory instability).

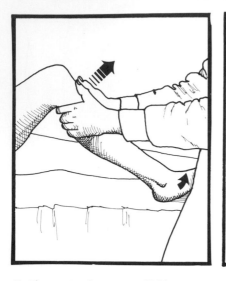

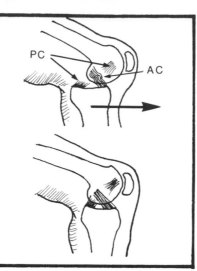

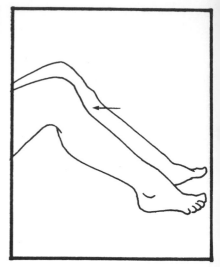

65. *The anterior drawer test:* (3) Next, turn the foot in to 30° internal rotation and repeat. If the lateral tibial condyle subluxes forwards, it suggests the presence of a rotatory instability of that pattern (antero-lateral rotational instability).

66. *The anterior drawer test:* (4) Beware of the following fallacy: a tibia *already* displaced backwards as a result of a posterior cruciate ligament tear may give a false positive in this test. Check by inspection prior to testing (see also 67).

67. *Posterior tibial displacement or instability:* Rupture, detachment or stretching of the posterior cruciate ligament may permit the tibia to sublux backwards, frequently giving rise to a striking deformity of the knee which allows the diagnosis to be made on inspection alone.

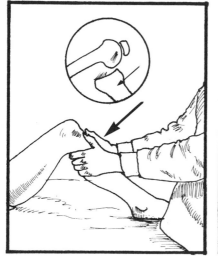

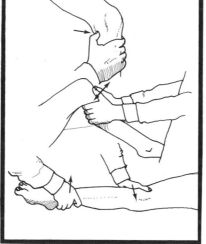

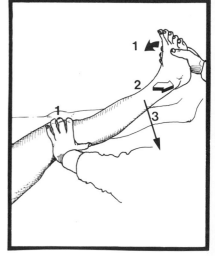

68. *Posterior drawer test:* Flex the knee to 80° and sit close to the foot to steady it. Attempt to jerk the tibia backwards. Displacement more than the other side suggests instability, and if substantial (say 1 cm or more) rupture of the posterior cruciate ligament is very likely to be present. Backward displacement of the lateral tibial condyle by a greater amount than the medial may occur in so-called postero-lateral rotatory insufficiency.

69. *Assessing tibial subluxations* (rotatory or torsional instabilities): (1) Look for medial or lateral tenderness or oedema. (2) Perform the drawer tests noting variations. (3) Test for laxity on valgus stress (usually positive in anterior subluxation of the medial tibial condyle). (4) Test for laxity on varus stress (usually positive when the lateral tibial condyle subluxes forwards or backwards. (5) Carry out tests 70–73.

70. *MacIntosh test for anterior subluxation of the lateral tibial condyle:* Fully extend the knee while holding the foot in internal rotation (1). Apply a valgus stress (2). In this position, if instability is present, the tibia will be in the subluxed position. Now flex the knee (3): reduction should occur at about 30° with an obvious jerk.

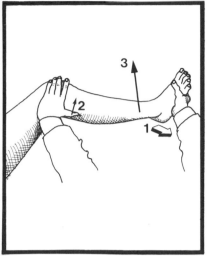

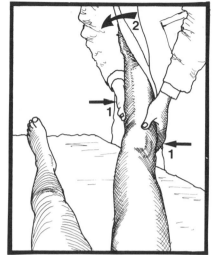

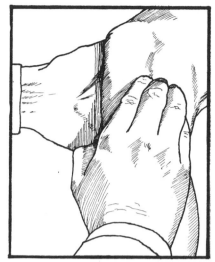

71. *Losee test for anterior subluxation of the lateral tibial condyle:* The patient should be completely relaxed, with no tension in the hamstrings. Apply a valgus force to the knee (1) at the same time pushing the fibular head anteriorly (2). The knee should be partly flexed. Now extend the joint (3). As full extension is reached, a dramatic clunk will occur as the lateral tibial condyle subluxes forwards (if rotatory instability is present). Note: the patient should relate this to the sensations experienced in activity.

72. *Modified jerk test for anterior subluxation of the lateral tibial condyle:* Grasp the foot between the arm and the chest, and apply a valgus stress (1); lean over to rotate the foot internally (2). Now flex the knee. If the test is positive, and because the tibia is firmly held, the lateral *femoral* condyle will appear to jerk anteriorly. Now extend the knee, and as the tibia subluxes, the femoral condyle will appear to jerk backwards.

73. *The menisci:* (1) Look for tenderness in the joint line, and test for a springy block to full extension. These two signs in association with evidence of quadriceps wasting are the most *consistent and reliable signs* of a torn meniscus.

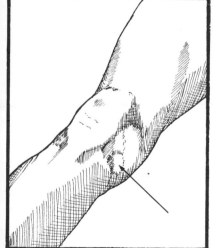

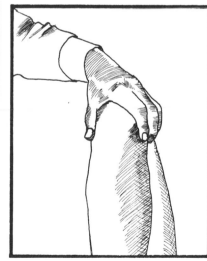

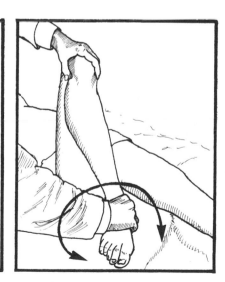

74. *The Menisci:* (2) In recent injuries, look for tell-tale oedema in the joint line.

75. *The Menisci:* (3) *Posterior lesions:* Fully flex the knee and place the thumb and index along the joint line. The palm of the hand should rest on the patella. You are now in a position to be able to locate any clicks emanating from the joint.

76. *The Menisci:* (4) *Posterior lesions:* Sweep the heel round in a U-shaped arc, looking and feeling for clicks from the joint accompanied by pain. Watch the patient's face, not the knee, while carrying out this test.

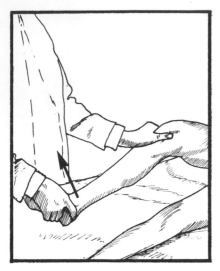

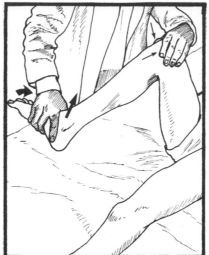

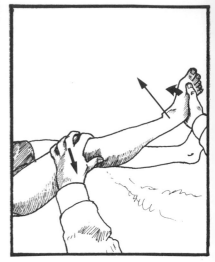

77. *The Menisci:* (5) *Anterior lesions:* Press the thumb firmly into the joint line at the medial side of the patellar ligament. Now extend the joint. Repeat on the other side of the ligament. A click, accompanied by pain, is found in anterior meniscus lesions.

78. *The Menisci:* (6) *McMurray manoeuvre for the medial meniscus:* Place the thumb and index along the joint line to detect any clicks. Flex the leg fully; externally rotate the foot, abduct the leg, and extend the joint smoothly.

79. *The Menisci:* (7) *McMurray manoeuvre for the lateral meniscus:* Repeat the last test with the foot internally rotated and the leg adducted. Use the hand to pick up any clicks accompanied by pain. A grating sensation is felt in degenerative lesions.

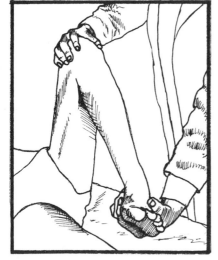

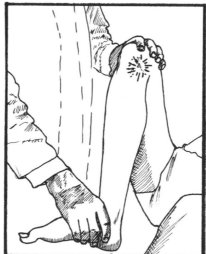

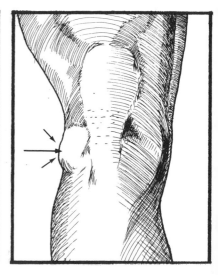

80. *The Menisci:* (8) If any clicks are detected, the normal limb should be examined to help eliminate symptomless, non-pathological clicks which may be arising from tendons or other soft tissues snapping over bony prominences (e.g. the biceps tendon over the femoral condyle).

81. *The Menisci:* (9) If a unilateral painful click is obtained, repeat the test with the sensing finger or thumb removed. The cause of the click, whether meniscus or tendon, may be visible on close inspection of the joint line.

82. *The Menisci:* (10) Meniscal cysts lie in the joint line, feel firm on palpation, and are tender on deep pressure. Cysts of the menisci may be associated with tears. Lateral meniscus cysts are by far the commonest. Cystic swellings on the medial side are sometimes due to ganglions arising from the pes anserinus (insertion of sartorius, gracilis and semitendinosus).

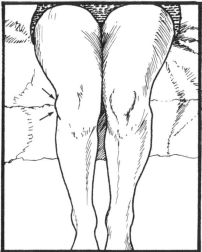

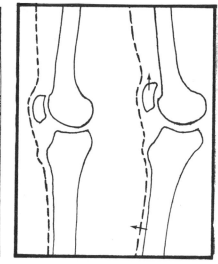

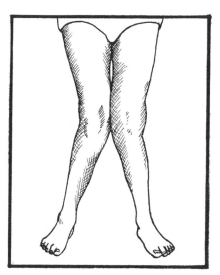

83. *The Patella:* (1) Examine both knees flexed over the end of the couch. This may show a torsional deformity of the femur or tibia, and a laterally placed patella.

84. *The Patella:* (2) Look for genu recurvatum and the position of the patella relative to the femoral condyles. A high patella (patella alta) is a predisposing factor in recurrent lateral dislocation of the patella.

85. *The Patella:* (3) Is there any knock knee deformity? Recurrent dislocation is commoner in women with this deformity.

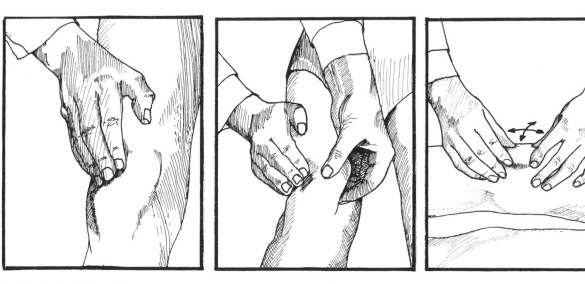

86. *The Patella:* (4) Look for tenderness over the anterior surface of the patella, and note if a tender, bi-partite ridge is present. Upper and lower pole tenderness occur in Sinding Larsen-Johannson disease and 'jumper's knee' (extensor apparatus traction injury).

87. *The Patella:* (5) Displace the patella medially and palpate its *articular* surface. Tenderness is found when the articular surface is diseased, e.g. in chondromalacia patellae. Repeat the test, displacing the patella laterally; 2/3 of the articular surface is thus accessible.

88. *The Patella:* (6) Test the *mobility* of the patella by moving it up and down and from side to side. Reduced mobility is found in retro-patellar arthritis. The quadriceps must be relaxed for adequate performance of this test.

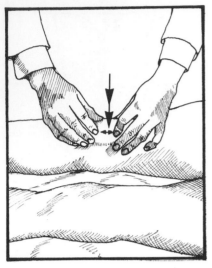

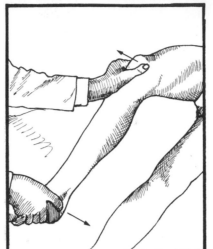

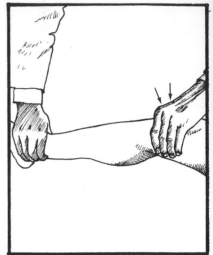

89. *The Patella:* (7) Move the patella proximally and distally, at the same time pressing it down hard against the femoral condyles. Pain is produced in chondromalacia patellae and retro-patellar arthritis.

90. *The Patella:* (8) *Apprehension test:* Try to displace the patella laterally while flexing the knee from the extended position. The patient will be apprehensive and try to stop the examination if there is a tendency to recurrent dislocation.

91. *Articular Surfaces:* (1) Place the palm of the hand over the patella, and the thumb and index along the joint line. Flex and extend the joint. The source of crepitations from damaged articular surfaces can then be detected. Compare one side with the other.

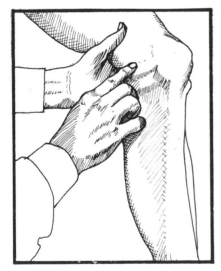

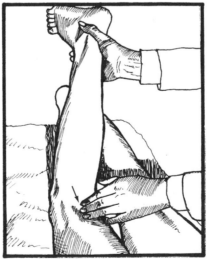

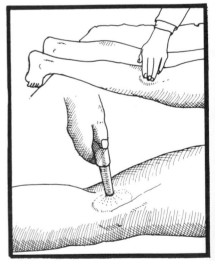

92. *Articular Surfaces:* (2) Apparent broadening of the joint and palpable exostoses occur commonly in osteo-arthritis. In this condition there is often laxity of the medial ligament if the medial compartment is extensively involved.

93. *Popliteal Region:* (1) All the previous tests have involved examination of the joint from the front. Examine the popliteal fossa by inspection and palpation. If the knee is flexed the roof of the fossa is relaxed, and deep palpation becomes possible.

94. *Popliteal Region:* (2) Semi-membranosus bursae become obvious when the knee is extended. Compare the sides. The bursa may be small at the time of examination, and transillumination is worth trying although not always positive. Note that semimembranosus bursae may be secondary to rheumatoid arthritis or other pathology in the joint.

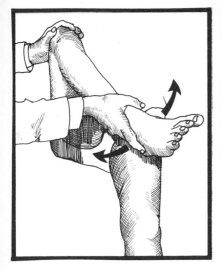

95. *The Hip:* Always examine the hip, especially in the presence of severe, undiagnosed pain, as hip pain is often referred to the knee joint. The hip may be screened by testing rotation at 90° flexion, noting pain or restriction of movements.

96. *Radiographs:* (1) Normal A-P radiograph of the knee.

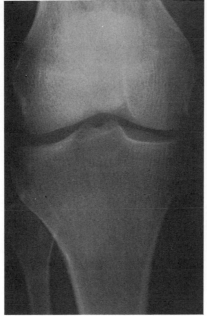

97. *Radiographs:* (2) Normal lateral radiograph of the knee.

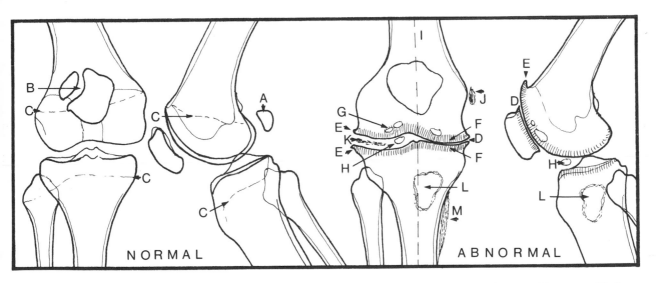

98. *Radiographs:* (3) The standard views are the non-weight-bearing A-P and lateral. *Do not mistake* (A) the normal inconstant fabella for a loose body, (B) bi-partite patella for fracture (this anomaly affects the outer quadrants), (C) epiphyseal lines for fracture. *Examine the articular margins* for (D) joint space narrowing (indicating cartilage loss), (E) lipping, (F) marginal sclerosis, (G) cysts, (H) loose bodies, varus or valgus (D–H common in O-A). Look for alterations in bone texture (e.g. in Paget's disease, rheumatoid arthritis, osteomalacia, infections). *Note* abnormal calcifications as in (J) Pellegrini-Stieda disease, (K) calcified meniscus and pseudo-gout. *Note bone defects and areas of periosteal reaction* (L, M), suggesting bone tumour or infection.

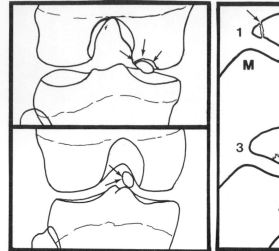

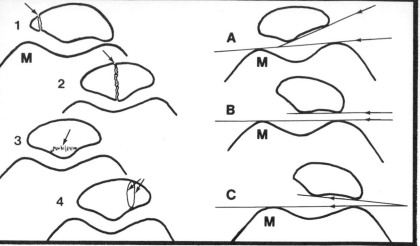

99. *Radiographs:* (4) Intercondylar radiographs are often of help in confirming the diagnosis of osteochondritis dissecans, as they show the common sites, especially in the medial femoral condyle. They are also of value in locating loose bodies.

100. *Radiographs:* (5) Where the patella is suspect, a tangential (skyline) view should be obtained. This may show (1) a marginal (medial) osteochondral fracture, common in recurrent dislocation of the patella, (2) other fractures, (3) occasionally, evidence of chondromalacia patellae, (4) bi-partite patella. A 20° projection (knee flexed to 20°, X-ray beam parallel to the tibia, film at right angles to the beam) may help in diagnosing recurrent dislocation. Draw tangents as shown. The angle is open laterally in 97% of normal subjects (A), but (B) the tangents are parallel (80%) or (C) open medially (20%) in those suffering from recurrent dislocation of the patella.

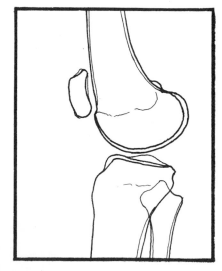

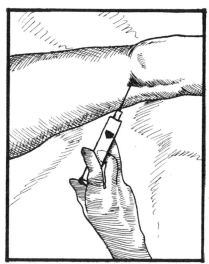

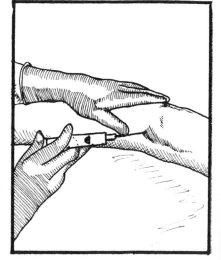

101. *Radiographs:* (6) Again in suspected recurrent dislocation of the patella, the lateral projection should be taken with the knee weight-bearing and held in full extension. This may confirm the presence of a highly placed and susceptible patella.

102. *Aspiration:* (1) Aspirate the knee (a) in the presence of a tense haemarthrosis or (b) to obtain specimens for bacteriology in suspected infections. Begin with full aseptic precautions by raising a skin weal with local anaesthetic just above and lateral to the patella.

103. *Aspiration:* (2) Infiltrate the tissues more deeply down to the level of the synovial membrane of the suprapatellar pouch.

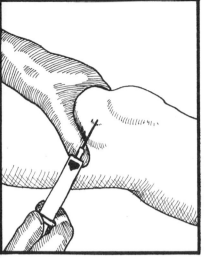
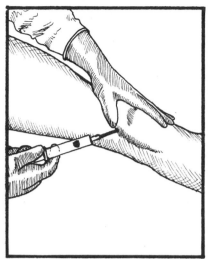
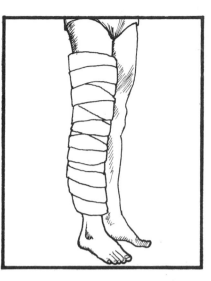
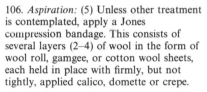

104. *Aspiration:* (3) Unless the knee is very tense, squeeze fluid from the upper limits of the suprapatellar pouch to float the patella forwards before inserting the aspiration needle.

105. *Aspiration:* (4) Squeeze the superior aspect and sides of the joint during the terminal stages of aspiration to empty the joint. Seal with Nobecutane and apply a sterile dressing.

106. *Aspiration:* (5) Unless other treatment is contemplated, apply a Jones compression bandage. This consists of several layers (2–4) of wool in the form of wool roll, gamgee, or cotton wool sheets, each held in place with firmly, but not tightly, applied calico, domette or crepe.

11 The Tibia

Common causes of pain in the anterior aspect of the lower leg

Note: Knock-knee and bow leg deformities are included with the knee-joint.

Osteitis of the tibia

Osteitis of the tibia occurs predominantly in children, with or without a history of previous trauma or sore throat. Pain is intense, tenderness is acute and initially well localised over the metaphyseal area and there is inability to weight-bear. There is systemic upset with fever and tachycardia, and often but not always a polymorph leucocytosis. Admission and investigation with repeated blood cultures is essential. Radiographs of the tibia are initially normal. When this condition is suspected, it is customary to administer a broad spectrum antibiotic, effective against the pencicillin resistant *Staphylococcus*, and in large doses to achieve adequate bone levels, prior to the results of blood culture. Splintage of the affected area is often helpful, and in proven cases antibiotics are administered for 4 weeks. Surgical drainage is seldom necessary and is avoided unless failure of response to antibiotics, profound toxicity and spread of the infection make it essential.

Cellulitis from insect stings, small wounds and abrasions and hair follicle infections may sometimes cause difficulty in diagnosis.

Low grade osteitis of the tibia (Brodie's abscess) may give rise to chronic upper tibial pain.

Bone tumours

The tibia is a common site for many primary bone tumours, so that radiographic examination of the tibia is essential in any case of undiagnosed leg pain.

Anterior tibial compartment syndrome

In this condition pain in the front of the leg is usually preceded by intense (usually athletic) activity. Oedema and swelling within the confines of the anterior compartment produce ischaemia, and eventually necrosis of muscle. The leg is diffusely swollen and tender, and the skin has a glossy appearance. Tibialis anterior and extensor hallucis longus are first affected, with weakness and later inability to

156

extend the ankle and great toe. The dorsalis pedis pulse may be absent, and there may be sensory loss in the first web space from ischaemic changes in the deep peroneal nerve. Immediate surgical decompression of the anterior tibial compartment is essential if muscle necrosis is to be avoided.

Stress fracture of the tibia

In this condition, the onset of leg pain may be sudden or less acute. There is sharply localised bone tenderness and overlying oedema. Radiographic demonstration of the hair line fracture may be difficult, and with persistent pain repeated examination is essential. In many cases the diagnosis may not be firmly established until a small area of tell-tale callus is showing. The condition is also common in Paget's disease where, of course there is an easily identifiable radiological abnormality.

Medial tibial syndrome

Pain on the medial side of the shin in sportsmen (shin splints) may be severe, and gives rise to tenderness along the postero-medial border of the lower part of the shin. In a number of cases the symptoms may arise from stress fractures of the tibia, but in others the pathology is less clear. Where symptoms are of a chronic nature, and fracture has been excluded, division of the attachments of the crural fascia may give relief.

Tabes dorsalis

Severe pain in the shins (lightning pains) is common in the tabes dorsalis. Usually other criteria are present (e.g. Argyll-Robertson pupils) and serological tests confirm the diagnosis.

Common causes of pain in the posterior aspect of the lower leg

1. *'Ruptured plantaris tendon'*. Sudden pain in the calf during activity with diffuse tenderness in the upper and outer part of the calf is now regarded as being due to tearing of muscle fibres of soleus or gastrocnemius rather than injury to the plantaris muscle. Pain often persists for several months and a period of plaster immobilisation is often helpful in relieving pain in the acute initial stages.

2. *Thrombo-phlebitis*. Thrombosis in the superficial veins of the calf with local inflammatory changes is a common cause of recurrent calf pain and the presence of tenderness and other inflammatory signs along the course of a calf vein make diagnosis easy. Thrombosis in the deep veins is often silent, and its importance in the post-operative situation is well known.

3. *Other causes of posterior leg pain*. Pain in the calf is common in patients suffering from prolapsed intervertebral discs. Claudication pain is a feature of vascular insufficiency and spinal stenosis. Lesions of the foot and ankle which lead to protective muscle spasm on standing and walking frequently give rise to marked calf and leg pain.

Deformities of the tibia

Alteration in the normal curvature of the tibia is not uncommon and may be a cause for complaint. The bone may curve convex laterally (tibial bowing), convex anteriorly (tibial kyphosis) or undergo a rotational deformity (tibial torsion). Deformities of these types are particularly likely to occur in infants and young children when the immature bone may yield under the weight of a relatively heavy child. In the majority of cases no other cause is apparent and spontaneous correction by the time the child reaches the age of 6 is the rule. Nevertheless rickets and other osteodystrophies must be excluded and continuous observation is essential.

Pseudarthrosis of the tibia is a rare congenital abnormality of the tibia which leads to progressive tibial kyphosis. The tibia becomes progressively thinner and undergoes spontaneous fracture which proceeds to non-union. It is particularly resistant to treatment. The diagnosis is made on the radiographic findings.

In the adult, deformity of the tibia may be seen following rickets in childhood, mal-united fractures, Paget's disease and syphilis.

Guide to commoner causes of leg pain

In children	Osteitis or other infections
	Bone tumour
Adolescents and young adults	Stress fracture tibia
	Bone tumours (especially osteoid osteoma, osteoclastoma, osteosarcoma)
	Brodie's abscess
	Anterior compartment syndrome
	Shin splints
Adults	PID and spinal stenosis
	Vascular insufficiency
	Thrombo-phlebitis
	Paget's disease
	'Ruptured plantaris tendon'
	Painful conditions of the foot
	Syphilis
	Bone tumours

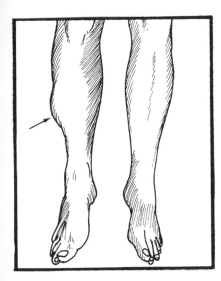

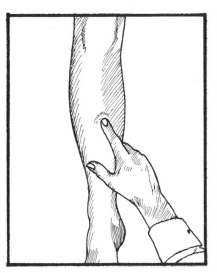

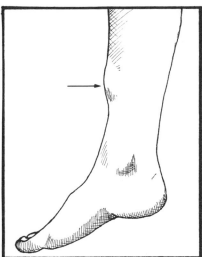

1. *Inspection* (1) *Soft tissue swelling:* Note the site and extent of any swelling. In the case of oedema, note particularly if bilateral (suggesting a general rather than a local cause). Unilateral leg oedema in women over 40 is a common sign of intrapelvic neoplasm.

2. *Inspection* (2) *Localised oedema:* Localised oedema is common over inflammatory lesions and stress fractures.

3. *Inspection* (3) *Local bone swelling:* This is suggestive of neoplasm (e.g. osteoid osteoma) or old fracture. Multiple or single exostoses commonly occur in the tibia in diaphyseal aclasis. Thickening of the ends of the tibia is seen in rickets, and osteo-arthritis.

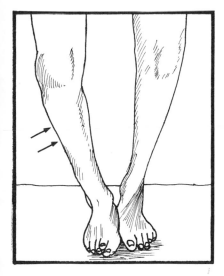

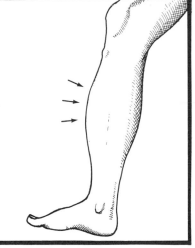

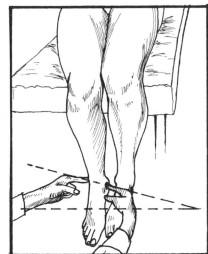

4 *Inspection* (4) *General bone thickening:* Extensive thickening of bone is characteristic of Paget's disease and long standing osteitis. In the latter case there are usually other signs such as scarring or sinuses.

5. *Inspection* (5) *Tibial shape:* Note any abnormal anterior curvature, possibly secondary to Paget's disease, mal-united fracture, syphilis or rickets. Rickets affects the distal half of both tibia and fibula, and there are associated lateral and torsional deformities.

6. *Tibial torsion:* (1) Flex the legs over the edge of the examination couch. The tibial tubercles must face directly forwards. Place the index fingers over the malleoli. The medial malleolus normally lies in front of the lateral 20° to the coronal plane).

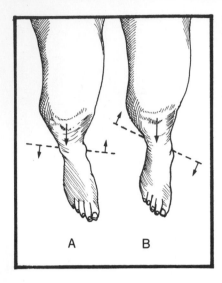

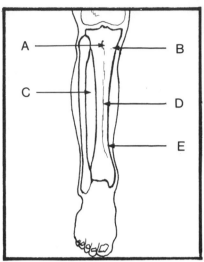

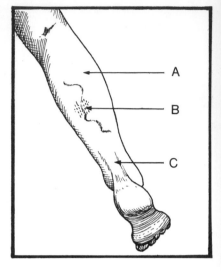

7. *Tibial torsion:* (2) (A) Medial torsional deformity (a decrease in the angle) is associated with flat foot and intoeing. (B) Lateral torsional deformity (an increase in the angle) is seen in pes cavus.

8. *Tenderness* (1) At the front, tenderness is characteristically sited in the following:
(A) Osgood-Schlatter's disease.
(B) Brodie's abscess, osteitis.
(C) Anterior tibial compartment syndrome.
(D) Stress fracture.
(E) Shin splints.

9. *Tenderness* (2) At the back of the leg, tenderness is characteristically situated in the following: (A) 'Ruptured plantaris tendon' syndrome. (B) Over varicosities in superficial thrombo-phlebitis. (C) Over the tendo-calcaneus in partial tears and complete ruptures.

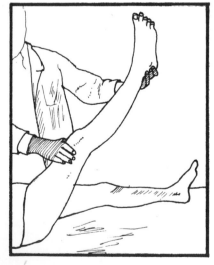

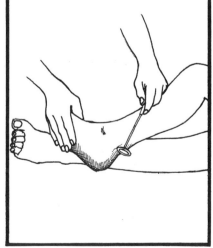

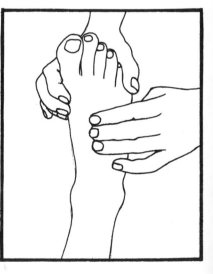

10. *Screening tests* (1) The following tests should be carried out in the investigation of any case of leg pain. The straight leg raising test (see *Lumbar Spine* 27) should be carried out. In many cases pain in the leg below the knee is referred from the spine.

11. *Screening tests* (2) The lower limb reflexes should be elicited, and if suggested, the pupils for reaction to light and accommodation. Lower leg pain is a common symptom of late syphilis.

12. *Screening tests* (3) The peripheral pulses should be sought (see also *Foot* 56). Ischaemia is an extremely common cause of leg pain.

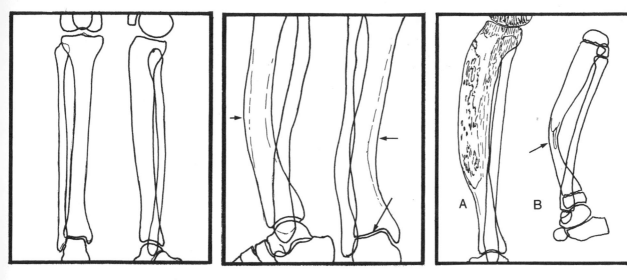

13. *Radiographs* (1) The standard films are an A–P and lateral which include both ends of tibia and fibula. For better visualisation of a suspect area, localised views are required. Tomography is sometimes of additional help especially in evaluating cystic defects.

14. *Radiographs* (2) Begin by noting the general shape of the bones, their texture and mineralisation. For example, in late rickets there is deformity following weight-bearing in the phase of bone softening. Note angulation of the plane of the ankle (pre-disposing to O–A).

15. *Radiographs* (3) Deformity is common in Paget's disease (A) where there is disturbance of form and texture, and sometimes sarcomatous change. In pseud-arthrosis of the tibia (B) there is local thinning and angulation progressing to dissolution, the fibula remaining normal.

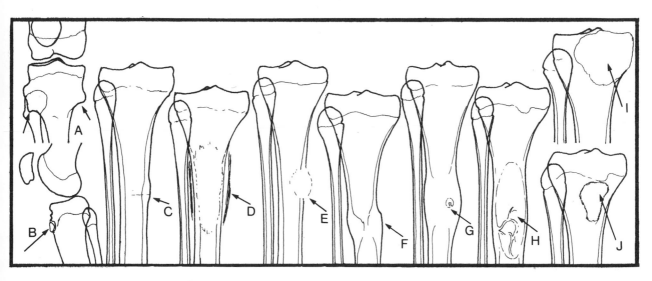

16. *Radiographs* (4) Note any localised deformity such as in (A) diaphyseal aclasis (often several bones affected), (B) Osgood-Schlatter's disease, (C) localised periosteal reaction in the region of a stress fracture, (D) more extensive sub-periosteal new bone formation in the later stages of osteitis, or at the site of a bone tumour. Note (E) cortical bone destruction suggesting a lytic neoplasm or infection. Localised thickening of bone is seen after a healed fracture (F) or again at a tumour site (e.g. in osteoid osteoma where there is often a central nidus). (G) Examine the cavity and ends of the bone for space occupying lesions such as (H) unicameral bone cyst occurring in the shaft, (I) osteoclastoma occurring in the epiphysis and (J) Brodie's abscess in the metaphysis.

12 The Ankle

Note that a careful examination of the foot is often also required in the investigation of many ankle complaints.

Soft tissue injuries of the ankle

Soft tissue injuries of the ankle are extremely common and in the severer cases difficult to differentiate from undisplaced Pott's fractures. Radiographic examination is essential in all but the most minor lesions, and is also necessary where symptoms are persistent. When fracture has been excluded after a significant injury a diagnosis has still to be made, as this manifestly affects treatment.

Injuries of the lateral ligament

The lateral ligament is damaged in inversion injuries. In an incomplete tear, some fibres only are ruptured (ankle sprain). Treatment is then symptomatic and a full early recovery can be expected. When the ligament is completely torn or detached from the fibula, the talus is free to tilt in the mortice of the tibia and fibula. If the lateral ligament fails to heal, chronic instability of the ankle results. If this injury is diagnosed, it should be treated by operative repair or prolonged immobilisation in plaster.

Inferior tibio-fibular ligaments

When the foot is dorsiflexed the distal end of the fibula moves laterally as it is engaged by the wedge-shaped upper articular surface of the talus. This movement is restricted by the inferior tibio-fibular ligaments, and to a lesser extent the interosseous membrane. Damage to these structures may lead to lateral displacement of the fibula and lateral drift of the talus (diastasis). In treatment, the talus must be realigned with the tibia, and any fibular displacement reduced. This reduction may be held by cross screwing of the fibula to the tibia, or by plaster fixation.

Medial ligament

The medial ligament is immensely strong and if stressed in ankle joint injuries generally avulses the medial malleolus rather than itself tearing. Nevertheless tears do occur, and are seen particularly in conjunction with lateral malleolar fractures. Meticulous reduction of any associated fracture is essential, and operative repair may be required.

Achilles tendon

Sudden plantar flexion of the foot may rupture the Achilles tendon, especially when it is weakened as a result of the degenerative changes seen in middle age. Surgical repair may be carried out, although in most cases excellent results may be achieved by conservative management in plaster.

Other common conditions seen round the ankle

Tenosynovitis

Inflammatory changes in the tendon sheaths behind the malleoli may give rise to pain at the sides of the ankle joint. Tenosynovitis may follow unusual activity or be associated with degenerative changes, flat foot or rheumatoid arthritis. There is puffy swelling in the line of the tendons, with tenderness extending often for several centimetres along their length. Tibialis posterior and peroneous longus are most frequently involved, and stretching these structures by forced inversion and eversion of the foot gives rise to pain. Spontaneous rupture is not uncommon. Symptoms generally respond to immobilisation for short periods in a below-knee walking plaster.

Footballer's ankle

Illocalised pain in the front of the ankle may follow repeated incidents of forced plantar-flexion of the foot which result in tearing of the anterior capsule of the ankle joint. This is found to occur frequently in footballers where this form of stress is common. Calcification in the resulting areas of avulsion and haemorrhage lead to the appearance of characteristic exostoses in lateral radiographic projections of the ankle.

Osteochondritis of the talus

Although rather uncommon, this condition, which is seen most frequently in adolescents and young men, may give disabling pain in the ankle. The diagnosis is made on the radiographic findings, although the site of the pain and local tenderness over the upper articular surface of the talus may lead one to suspect it. If loose bodies are produced, they must be excised. The treatment of the local lesion in principle follows that of osteochondritis dissecans of the knee.

Snapping peroneal tendons

This is an uncommon cause of ankle pain and is due to tearing of the peroneal retinaculum. The patient complains of a clicking sensation in the ankle and is usually able to demontrate the peroneal tendons riding ovr the lateral malleolus. The treatment is by surgical reconstruction of the retinaculum.

Osteo-arthritis

Primary osteo-arthritis of the ankle is rare. Osteo-arthritis is sometimes seen secondary to Pott's fracture, avascular necrosis of the talus, or osteochondritis of the talus.

Rheumatoid arthritis

Rheumatoid arthritis of the ankle is not uncommon, but is seldom seen as a primary manifestation of the disease, so that diagnosis seldom presents difficulty.

Tuberculosis

Tuberculous infections of the ankle joint are now rare in Great Britain. There is swelling of the joint, wasting of the calf, and the usual signs of inflammation. The patient develops a painful limp, and as the joint is comparatively superficial, sinus formation is common at a comparatively early stage.

Shortening of the Achilles tendon (tendo calcaneus)

Shortening of the Achilles tendon results in plantar-flexion of the foot and clumsiness of gait as the heel fails to reach the ground. The more severe degrees of Achilles tendon shortening are accompanied by inversion of the heel. In many cases flexion of the knee, by taking the tension off the gastrocnemius, will permit dorsiflexion of the foot. Shortening of the Achilles tendon may occur as an apparently isolated condition with no obvious pre-disposing cause, but in a great many cases it is associated with congenital deformities of the foot or neurological disorders of which sub-clinical poliomyelitis is one of the commonest (for talipes deformities see *Foot* section). Occasionally it may result from ischaemic contracture of the calf muscles.

Guide to painful conditions round the ankle

History of recent injury   Sprain of lateral ligament

            Complete tear of lateral ligament

            (Pott's fracture, fracture of the fifth (metatarsal base)

            Diastasis

            Ruptured Achilles tendon (tendo calcaneus)

History of past injury   Complete tear of lateral ligament

            Secondary osteo-arthritis (e.g. previous Pott's fracture)

No history of injury   Osteochondritis tali

            Rheumatoid arthritis

            Primary osteo-arthritis

            Footballer's ankle

            Secondary osteo-arthritis (e.g. osteochondritis tali)

            Tenosynovitis

            Snapping peroneal tendons

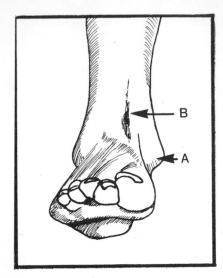

1. *Inspection* (1) Look for (A) deformity of shape, suggesting recent or old fracture, (B) sinus scars, suggesting old infection, particularly tuberculosis.

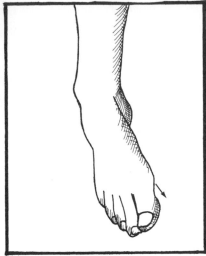

2. *Inspection* (2) Look for deformity of posture (e.g. plantar-flexion from short tendo calcaneus, talipes deformity (see *Foot* 1), ruptured tendo calcaneus or drop foot).

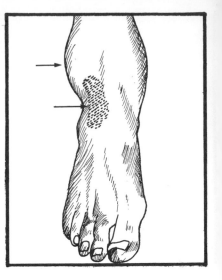

3. *Inspection* (3) Look for bruising, swelling or oedema. If there is any swelling, note if diffuse or localised. Note also if oedema is bilateral, suggesting a systemic rather than a local cause.

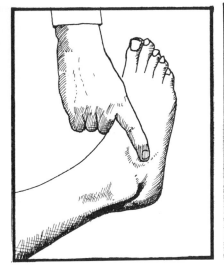

4. *Tenderness* (1) When there is tenderness localised over the malleoli following injury, radiographic examination is necessary to exclude fracture.

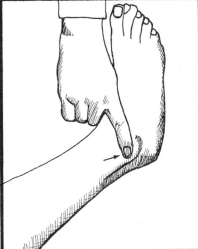

5. *Tenderness* (2) After inversion sprains, tenderness is often diffuse. Swelling, to begin with, lies in the line of the fasciculi of the lateral ligament.

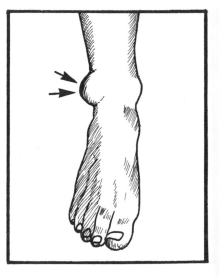

6. *Lateral ligament* (1) *Complete lateral ligament tear:* Swelling is rapid, and if seen within two hours of injury, is egg shaped and placed *over the lateral malleolus.*

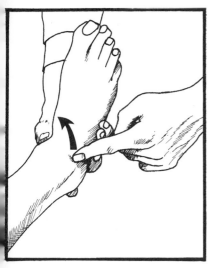

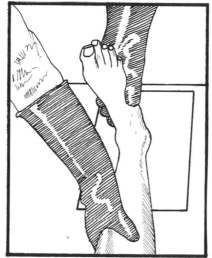

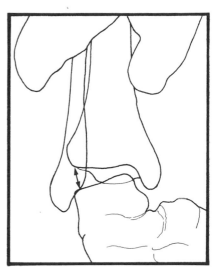

7. *Lateral ligament* (2) Stress test (for complete tears). Grasp the heel and forcibly invert the foot, feeling for any opening up of the lateral side of the ankle between tibia and talus.

8. *Lateral ligament* (3) If in doubt, have a radiograph taken while the foot is forcibly inverted.

9. *Lateral ligament* (4) If tilting of the talus in the ankle mortice is demonstrated, repeat the examination on the other side, and compare the films.

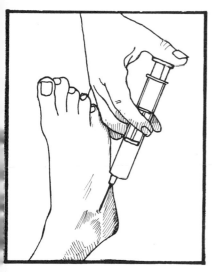

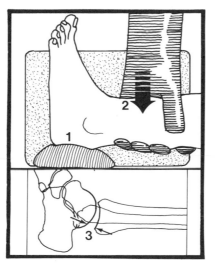

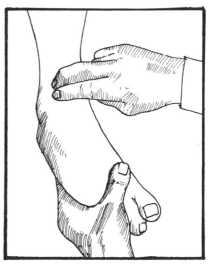

10. *Lateral ligament* (5) If the injury is fresh and painful, the examination may be more readily permitted after the injection of 15–20 ml of ½ per cent lignocaine widely in the region of the lateral ligament.

11. *Lateral ligament* (6) Instability may sometimes follow tears of the anterior talo-fibular portion only of the lateral ligament, and may be confirmed by radiographs after local anaesthesia. Support the heel on a sandbag (1) and press firmly downwards on the tibia (2) for 30 seconds up to exposure. A gap between the talus and tibia of >6mm is regarded as pathological (3).

12. *Inferior tibio-fibular ligament* (1) In tears of this ligament (which has anterior and posterior components) tenderness is present over the ligament just above the line of the ankle joint.

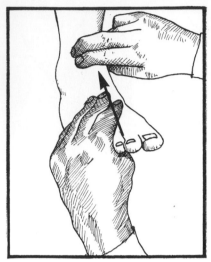

13. *Inferior tibio-fibular ligament* (1) In tears of the ligament, pain is produced by dorsiflexion of the foot which displaces the fibula laterally.

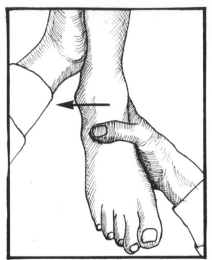

14. *Inferior tibio-fibular ligament* (3) Grasp the heel and try to move the talus directly laterally in the ankle mortice. Lateral displacement indicates a tear of the ligament.

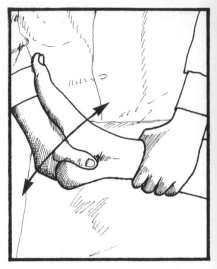

15. *Movements* (1) First confirm that the ankle is mobile, and that any apparent movement is not arising in the mid-tarsal or more distal joints. Firmly grasp the foot proximal to the mid-tarsal joint; try to produce dorsiflexion and plantar-flexion.

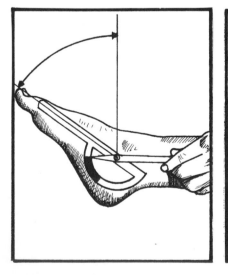

16. *Movements* (2) Measure *plantar-flexion* from the zero position. This reference is at right angles to the line of the leg. *Normal range:* 55°

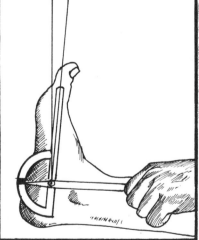

17. *Movements* (3) Measure the range of *dorsiflexion*. Always compare the sides. *Normal range:* 15°

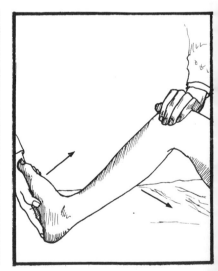

18. *Movements* (4) If dorsiflexion is restricted, bend the knee. If this restores a normal range, the Achilles tendon is tight. If it makes no difference, joint pathology (such as osteoarthritis, rheumatoid arthritis or infection) is the likely cause.

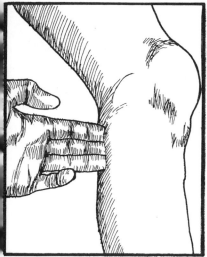

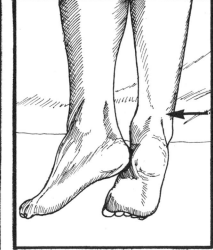

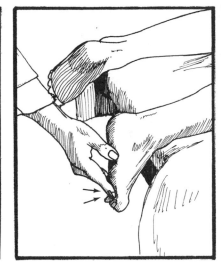

19. *Movements* (5) If there is loss of active dorsiflexion (drop foot) a full neurological examination is required. The commonest causes are stroke, old polio, prolapsed lumbar discs and local lesions of the common peroneal (lateral popliteal) nerve.

20. *Tendo calcaneus* (Achilles tendon) (1) The patient should be prone, with the feet over the edge of the couch. Defects in the contour of the tendon may be obvious. Note any enlargement of the bursae related to the tendon.

21. *Tendo calcaneus* (2) Test the power of plantar-flexion by asking the patient to press the foot against your hand. Compare one side with the other, and note the shape of each contracting calf and the prominence of each tendon.

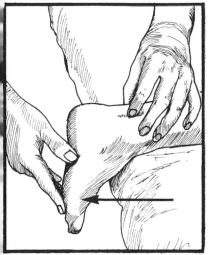

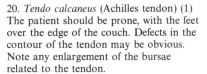

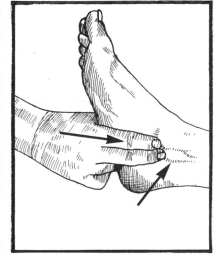

22. *Tendo calcaneus* (3) Palpate the tendon while the patient continues resisted plantarflexion. Compare the sides. Any gap in the tendon (ruptured tendo calcaneus) should be obvious.

23. *Teno-synovitis* (1) *Medial:* Look for tenderness along the line of the long flexor tendons. Tenderness is usually diffuse and linear in pattern. Note any local thickening.

24. *Teno-synovitis* (2) Look for synovitis in relation to the flexor tendons. There may be obvious swelling. Demonstrate excess fluid by milking the tendon sheaths proximally.

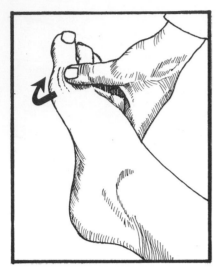

25. *Teno-synovitis* (3) Plantar flex and evert the foot. This may produce pain where teno-synovitis involves the tendon of tibialis posterior.

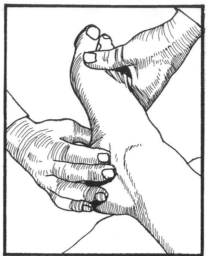

26. *Teno-synovitis* (4) With the foot held in the plantar flexed and everted position, look for tenderness or gaps (spontaneous rupture) in the line of the tendon of tibialis posterior. Spontaneous rupture is seen most frequently in flat foot and rheumatoid arthritis.

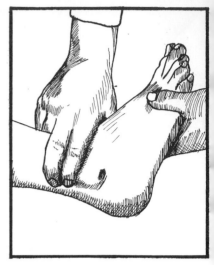

27. *Teno-synovitis* (5) *Lateral:* Examine the peroneal tendons for tenderness and the presence of excess synovial fluid in their sheaths.

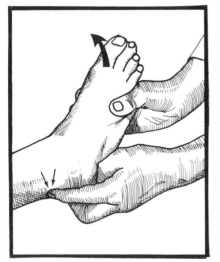

28. *Teno-synovitis* (6) Force the foot into plantar-flexion and inversion. This will give rise to pain and increase tenderness along the line of the peroneal tendons.

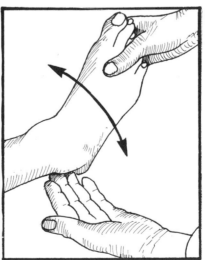

29. *Teno-synovitis* (7) Feel for crepitations along the line of the tendon sheaths behind both malleoli as the foot is swung backwards and forward between inversion and eversion.

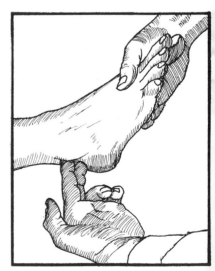

30. *Peroneal tendons:* Lightly palpate the peroneal tendons with the fingers; look and feel for displacement of the tendons as the patient everts the foot against light resistance. Displacement occurs in the condition known as 'snapping peroneal tendons'.

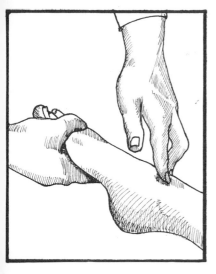

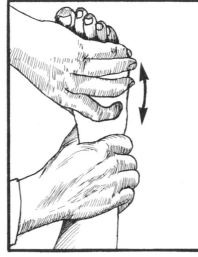

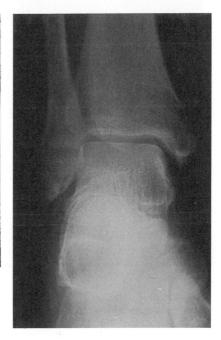

31. *Articular surfaces* (1) Forcibly plantar-flex the foot to allow palpation of part of the articular surface of the talus. Tenderness occurs in arthritic conditions, and in osteochondritis of the talus. A tender exostosis may be palpable in footballer's ankle.

32. *Articular surfaces* (2) Place a hand across the front of the ankle and passively dorsiflex and plantar flex the foot. Crepitations suggest articular damage.

33. *Radiographs* (1) Normal A-P radiograph of the ankle.

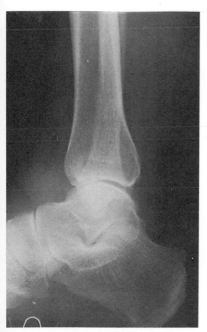

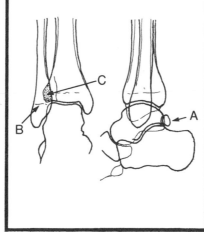

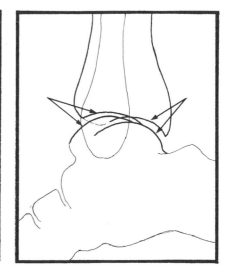

34. *Radiographs* (2) Normal lateral radiograph of the ankle.

35. *Radiographs* (3) The standard views are the A-P projection and lateral. Do not mistake (A) the common os trigonum accessory bone and (B) the epiphyseal line of the fibula for fractures. The amount of tibio-fibular overlap (C) is dependent on positioning and any diastasis.

36. *Radiographs* (4) The articular margins of tibia and talus should appear as two congruent circular arcs. If there is some difficulty in positioning which cannot be improved, four arcs will be seen. Two pairs should be congruent as shown. If not, there is a subluxation.

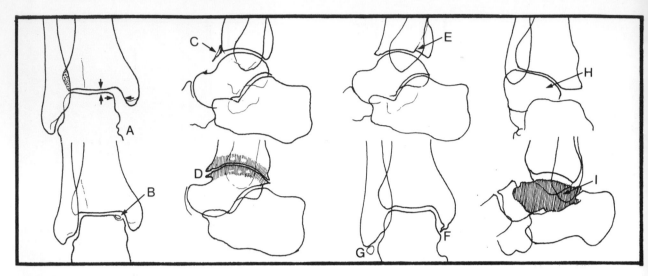

37. *Radiographs* (5) Examine the joint space. (A) Widening of the gap between talus and medial malleolus is suggestive of diastasis (compare with gap between upper surface of talus and the tibia). (B) Note the presence of any defects in the articular surface of the talus suggestive of osteochondritis tali. (C) Note the articular margins of the tibia—excrescences are found in footballer's ankle and (D) in osteo-arthritis where there is also joint narrowing and sclerosis. Note (E) any irregularity in the joint surfaces which may suggest previous injury. Look at the malleoli where deformity (F) or rounded shadows (G) suggest previous avulsion injuries. Distortion of the talus occurs in association with talipes deformities (H) and after injuries which have resulted in avascular necrosis (I). These may show increased bone density.

13 The Foot

Conditions commencing or seen first in childhood

Talipes equino varus

This is the commonest of the major congenital abnormalities affecting the foot, and all newly born children should be examined to exclude this condition. The deformity is a complex one; characteristically there is a varus deformity of the heel and adduction of the forefoot accompanied by some degree of plantar-flexion and inversion. Treatment in the form of corrective stretching of the foot and splintage must be started immediately if a good result is to be achieved. In some cases, especially when there is a delay in starting treatment, serial corrective plasters with or without surgery to some of the soft tissues involved may be required (e.g. lengthening of the Achilles tendon and division of the plantar fascia at the heel). In untreated cases the primary anomaly of soft tissue is followed by alteration in tarsal bone growth. In such cases, wedge excision of bone and fusion of the mid-tarsal and sub-talar joints is required to obtain a plantigrade foot (Dunn's arthrodesis, triple fusion).

When an incomplete correction has been obtained the commonest residual deformities seen in the older child and adult are persistent adduction of the forefoot, shortening of the Achilles tendon and some stunting in overall growth of the foot.

Talipes calcaneus

This is a much less common congenital abnormality of the foot in which the dorsum of the child's foot lies against the shin. There are frequently associated deformities of the sub-talar and mid-tarsal joints with the heel lying in the varus or valgus position (talipes calcaneo-varus, talipes calcaneo-valgus). Treatment in this condition by stretching and splintage is also carried out as soon as the diagnosis has been made.

Intoeing

After a child has commenced walking help may be sought because of intoeing (hen-toe gait). The feet may be internally rotated to such an extent that the child is constantly tripping and falling. Sometimes this may be due to torsional deformity of the tibiae, which should always be excluded, but more often is due to a postural deformity of the hips (internal rotation) or excessive anteversion of the femoral neck. The condition generally corrects spontaneously by the age of six. Continued observation is advised until correction occurs, but active treatment is seldom required.

Flat foot

The arches of the foot do not become fully formed until a child has been walking for some years; the young child's foot is normally flat. Failure of establishment of the arches leads to awkwardness of gait, rapid, uneven wear and distortion of the shoes, but seldom pain or other symptoms. Persistent flat foot may be associated with knock knees, torsional deformities of the tibiae and valgus deformities of the heel. Rarely it may result from an abnormal talus (vertical talus), or neuromuscular disorders of the limb (e.g. poliomyelitis, muscular dystrophies). In the majority of cases simple measures only are required (well fitting shoes, and sometimes supportive insoles, and physiotherapy). In the older child gross deformities may require surgery, which is dependent on the pathology (e.g. corrective sub-talar [Grice] fusion for severe valgus heels).

Pes cavus

Abnormally high longitudinal arches are produced by muscle imbalance which disturbs the forces controlling the formation and maintenance of the arches. In many cases there is a first metatarsal drop (an increase in the angle between the first metatarsal and the tarsus) and a varus deformity of the heel. Two distinct groups are seen: those in which sub-talar mobility is maintained, and those in which sub-talar movements are decreased or absent. A neurological abnormality should always be sought, and sometimes this may be obvious (e.g. spastic diplegia or old poliomyelitis). Many cases are associated with spina bifida occulta, which may be confirmed by clinical and radiological examination. Rarely fibrosis of the muscles of the posterior compartment of the leg from ischaemia may be the cause. In the more severe cases there is weakness of the intrinsic muscles of the foot, with clawing of the toes; the abnormal distrubition of weight in the foot leads to excessive callous formation under the metatarsal heads and the heel.

When the deformity is marked, surgery is indicated to relieve symptoms and lessen the chances of ultimate skin breakdown under the metatarsal heads. Where there is a varus deformity of the heel, correction of this defect alone may give good results; in some cases a wedge osteotomy of the distal tarsus or metatarsal bases is required to flatten the highly curved arch and improve the weight distribution in the foot. Where clawing of the toes is the most striking finding, proximal interphalangeal joint fusions of the toes or transplanting the flexor into the extensor tendons may be helpful.

Kohler's disease

This is an osteochondritis of the navicular occurring in children between the ages of 3 and 10. Pain of a mild character is centred over the medial side of the foot. Symptoms settle spontaneously over a few months and are not influenced by treatment.

Sever's disease

Chronic pain in the heel in children in the 6 to 12 age group generally arises from the calcaneal epiphysis which radiographically often shows increased density and fragmentation. The condition is usually referred to as Sever's disease, which although originally considered to be an osteochondritis is now believed to be due to a traction injury of the Achilles tendon insertion. Symptoms settle spontaneously without treatment.

Conditions affecting the adolescent foot

Hallux valgus

In adolescence, and particularly in girls where there is competition between the rapidly growing foot, tight stockings and often small, high heeled, unsuitable shoes, valgus deformity of the great toe first appears. In some cases a hereditary short and varus first metatarsal may contribute to the problem. As the deformity progresses, the drifting proximal phalanx of the great toe uncovers the metatarsal head, which presses against the shoe and leads to the formation of a protective bursa (bunion), often associated with recurrent episodes of inflammation (bursitis). Further lateral drift of the great toe results in crowding of the other toes; the great toe may pass over the second toe or more commonly the second toe may ride over it. The second toe may press against the toe cap of the shoe where there is little room for it, and develop painful callouses. Later the toe may dislocate at the metatarsophalangeal joint. The sesamoid bones under the first metatarsal head may be disturbed, leading to sharply localised pain under the first metatarsophalangeal joint. In the late stages of the condition, arthritic changes may develop in the metatarsophalangeal joint. More commonly, there is associated disturbance of the mechanics of the forefoot, leading to anterior metatarsalgia.

A number of surgical procedures are available to correct hallux valgus deformity. The most popular are: (a) fusion of the metatarsophalangeal joint in a corrected position, (b) Keller's arthroplasty (excision of the prominent part of the metatarsal head and removal of the basal portion of the proximal phalanx), (c) osteotomy of the first metatarsal neck (Mitchell operation), and (d) in early cases, simple excision of the prominent part of the metatarsal head may give relief.

Peroneal (spastic) flat foot

In adolescents (boys in particular) painful flat foot may be found in association with apparent spasm of the peroneal muscles. The foot is held in a fixed, everted position. Inversion of the foot is not permitted, and there is often marked disturbance of gait. The condition is frequently associated with ossification in a congenital cartilaginous bar bridging the calcaneus and navicular; this anomaly may be demonstrated radiologically. Surgery, in the form of excision of the bar, is now the normal treatment for this condition.

Exostoses

Apart from the first metatarsal head exposed in hallux valgus, several exostoses may give rise to trouble in adolescence.

1. *Calcaneal exostosis.* Prominence of the calcaneus above and to the sides of the Achilles tendon insertion may cause problems with friction against the counter of the shoe (blisters, callouses, difficulty in shoe fitting).
2. *Cuneiform exostosis.* An exostosis formed by lipping of the first metatarsal and medial cuneiform may cause similar difficulties.
3. *Fifth metatarsal head.* Prominence of the fifth metatarsal head may occur and is often associated with a varus deformity of the fifth toe (quinti varus).

All the above conditions are treated by local excision of the prominence.

4. *Fifth metatarsal base.* The base of the fifth metatarsal is sometimes enlarged and unduly prominent, especially in the narrow foot; it may sometimes cause pressure against the shoe, but surgical treatment is seldom required.

Conditions affecting the adult foot

Hallux rigidus

Primary osteo-arthritis of the M-P joint of the great toe often commences in adolescence and gives rise ultimately to pain and stiffness in this joint. It is commoner in males, and not associated with hallux valgus. Sometimes the toe is held in a flexed position (hallux flexus) and the proximal phalanx and metatarsal head are thickened following joint narrowing with circumferential exostosis formation. Treatment is usually by fusion or Keller's arthroplasty.

Adult flat foot

Gradual flattening of the medial longitudinal arch (incipient flat foot) may occur in those who spend much of the day on their feet. This is often associated with increase in body weight and the degenerative changes of ageing in the supporting structures of the arch. When these changes are rapid, they give rise to pain (medial foot strain). Secondary (tarsal) athritic changes may also give rise to pain in long standing flat foot and are associated with loss of movement in the foot (rigid flat foot). Where the mobility of the foot is preserved, flat foot may be symptom-free (mobile flat foot).

In the early stages, adult flat foot may be helped by weight reduction, physiotherapy and arch supports. In the later stages, surgical shoes with moulded insoles may be the most helpful measure.

Splay foot and anterior metatarsalgia

Widening of the foot at the level of the metatarsal heads is known as splay foot. This may occur as a variation in the normal pattern of foot growth, causing no difficulty apart from that of obtaining suitable footwear. Splay foot may also be seen in association with metatarsus primus varus, hallux valgus and pes cavus.

Anterior metatarsalgia (pain under the metatarsal heads) is particularly common in the middle-aged woman and is also often associated with some splaying of the forefoot. Symptoms may be triggered off by periods of excessive standing or increase in weight, and there is often a concurrent flattening of the medial longitudinal arch. Weakness of the intrinsic muscles is usually present so that there is a tendency to clawing of the toes; hyperextension of the toes at the M-P joints leads to exposure of the plantar surfaces of the metatarsal heads which give high spots of pressure against the underlying skin. In turn this produces pain and callous formation in the sole.

This pathological process is by far the commonest cause of forefoot pain, but in every case March fracture, Freiberg's disease, plantar digital neuroma and verruca pedis should be excluded.

The majority of cases of anterior metatarsalgia respond to skilled chiropodial measures, which include trimming of callouses and provision of supports—these distribute the weight-bearing loads more evenly on the metatarsal heads. Where there is much splaying of the forefoot and associated toe deformities, surgical shoes may be required. Where there is a marked hallux valgus deformity, an M-P joint fusion may improve the mechanics of the forefoot with relief of pain.

March fracture

This occurs in young adults and involves the second or less commonly the third and fourth metatarsals. The fracture usually follows a period of unaccustomed activity (there is no history of injury) and pain settles after 5 to 6 weeks on union of the fracture.

Freiberg's disease

This is an osteochondritis of the second metatarsal head associated with palpable deformity and pain. Pain may persist for 1 to 2 years and in severe cases excision of the metatarsal head may become necessary.

Plantar (digital) neuroma (Morton's metatarsalgia)

A neuroma situated on one of the plantar digital nerves just prior to its bifurcation at one of the toe clefts may give rise to piercing pain in the foot. It most commonly affects the plantar nerve running between the third and fourth metatarsal heads to the third web space, but any of the digital nerves may be affected. It most commonly occurs in women, particularly in the 25 to 45 age group, and is treated by excision of the affected nerve.

Verruca pedis (plantar warts)

Verrucae, thought to be viral in origin, are common in the metatarsal region, the great toe and the heel. They must be differentiated from callouses, and are usually treated by careful, local applications of caustic preparations such as salicylic acid, acetic acid and carbon dioxide snow.

Plantar fasciitis

Pain in the heel is a common complaint in the middle-aged and may be due to tearing of the calcaneal attachment of the plantar fascia following degenerative changes in its structure. Treatment is by the use of Sorbo-rubber pads in the heel of the shoe, physiotherapy in the form of ultrasound, or by the local infiltration of hydrocortisone.

Hammer toe, mallet toe

A flexion deformity of the proximal interphalangeal joint of a toe (hammer toe) may give rise to the formation of a troublesome corn on its dorsal surface. Treatment is by interphalangeal joint fusion. Flexion deformity of the distal interphalangeal joint gives pain from callous at the tip of the toe and pressure on the nail: treatment is by amputation of the distal phalanx.

The nail of the great toe

Ingrowing of the great toe nail gives rise to pain and a tendency to recurrent infection at the nail fold. If infection is not a problem, skilled chiropody treatment (e.g. by nail training using a prosthetic device) is usually successful.

Where infection is marked, avulsion of the nail to permit drainage and healing is often required. In chronic cases, ablation of the nail bed may be carried out to give a permanent cure.

Gross thickening and deformity of the nail (onychogryphosis) may also be treated by ablation of the nail bed or by regular chiropody.

Subungual exostosis, often a source of great pain, is treated by surgical removal of the exostosis.

Deformities of the nails may result from mycelial infections and are very resistant to treatment.

Irregularity of nail growth is a common feature of psoriasis and is usually associated with skin lesions elsewhere. There may be an accompanying psoriatic arthritis.

Rheumatoid arthritis

The foot is commonly involved in rheumatoid arthritis and the deformities are often multiple and severe. They frequently include pes planus, splay foot, hallux valgus, clawing of the toes and subluxation of the toes at the M-P joints. Anterior metatarsalgia is often marked. Sometimes a single deformity, such as a hammer toe, may be the main source of the patient's symptoms and may be amenable to a simple local surgical procedure. Where there are many deformities, the prescription of surgical shoes with moulded insoles may be the best treatment. Where there is gross crippling deformity, Fowler's operation, which is an arthroplasty of all the metatarsophalangeal joints combined with a plastic reconstruction of the metatarsal weight-bearing pad, is often helpful in the older patient; the best results may be obtained when the procedure is combined with fusion of the first M-P joint.

Gout

Gout classically affects the M-P joint of the great toe, but in severe cases the other M-P joints and even the tarsal joints are involved in the arthritic process. The treatment is mainly medical but surgical footwear may be required.

Tarsal tunnel syndrone

The posterior tibial nerve may become compressed as it passes beneath the flexor retinaculum into the sole of the foot, giving rise to paraesthesiae and burning pain in the sole of the foot and in the toes. The condition is uncommon, but is relieved by division of the flexor retinaculum.

Diagnosis of foot complaints

The following table lists the commonest disorders and relates them to the age groups in which they have the highest incidence.

	Heel pain	Pain on dorsal and medial side of foot	Great toe pain	Forefoot pain
Children	Sever's disease	Kohler's disease	Tight shoes and stockings Ingrowing toe nail	Verruca pedis
Adolescents	Calcaneal exostosis Bursitis	Cuneiform exostosis Peroneal flat foot	Early hallux rigidus Bunion Hallux valgus, nail problems	March fracture Freiberg's disease Pes cavus Verruca pedis
Adults	Plantar fasciitis	Flat foot Osteo-arthritis Rheumatoid arthritis	Hallux valgus and bunion Hallux rigidus Gout, nail problems	Anterior metatarsalgia Plantar neuroma Pes cavus Rheumatoid arthritis Gout Verruca pedis Tarsal tunnel syndrome

In assessing flat foot and pes cavus, the following table may be helpful:

	Factors in flat foot	Factors in pes cavus
Infants	'Normal foot' Vertical talus	In all age groups, this is due to muscle imbalance often from a neurological disorder, e.g.,
Children	Knock knees Valgus heels Neurological disturbance Torsional deformities of the tibia	spastic diplegia poliomyletis Freidrich's ataxia peroneal muscle atrophy spina bifida (usually occulta).
Adolescents	Continuation of childhood factors Peroneal flat foot	Many cases are associated with varus heels
Adults	Continuation of childhood factors Overweight, excessive standing Degenerative processes	

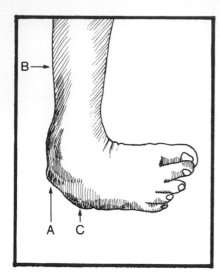

1. *Club Foot* (1) *Talipes eq. varus:* In the untreated case there is (A) persisting varus of the heel, (B) atrophy of the calf muscles, (C) callus where the child walks on the lateral border of the foot. It is commoner in males, may be bilateral, and may be associated with other anomalies.

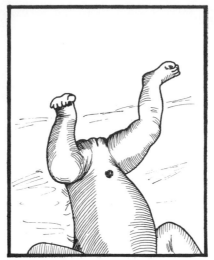

2. *Club Foot:* (2) The new born child often holds the foot in planter-flexion and inversion. First observe the child as it kicks to see if this position is maintained.

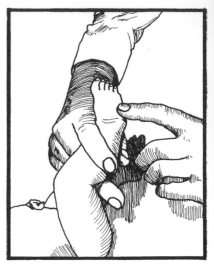

3. *Club Foot:* (3) If the child maintains the foot in the inverted position, support the leg and lightly scratch the side of the foot.

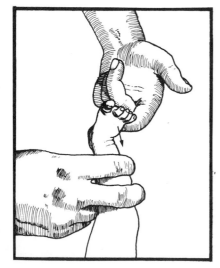

4. *Club Foot:* (4) In the normal foot the child will respond by dorsiflexion of the foot, eversion, and fanning of the toes. This reaction does not take place if the child has a talipes deformity.

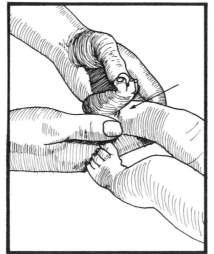

5. *Club Foot:* (5) If the child does not respond in a normal fashion, gently dorsiflex the foot. In the normal child, the foot can be brought into contact or close to the tibia without effort.

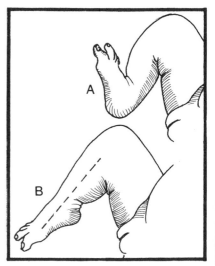

6. *Club Foot:* (6) (A) Note that in the less common talipes calcaneus deformity, the foot is held in a position of dorsiflexion. (B) Note that in the normal infant the foot can be plantar flexed to such a degree that the foot and tibia are in line.

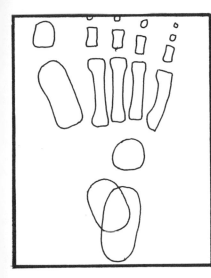

7. *Radiographs: A-P View:* (1) Interpretation is difficult due to the incompleteness of ossification. Centres for the talus, calcaneus, metatarsals, phalanges, and often the cuboid are present at birth. Begin by drawing a line through the long axis of the talus.

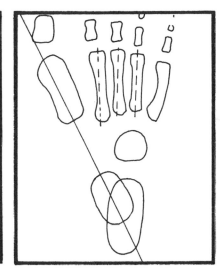

8. *Radiographs: A-P View:* (2) This line normally passes through the first metatarsal, or lies along its medial edge. Note also that the axes of the middle three metatarsals are roughly parallel. Now draw a second line through the long axis of the calcaneus.

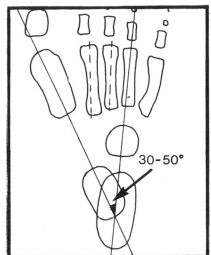

9. *Radiographs: A-P View:* (3) Note (A) the axial line of the calcaneus passes through or close to the fourth metatarsal. (B) The axes of the talus and calcaneus subtend an angle of 30°–50° (see 113 for radiographic appearance of vertical talus).

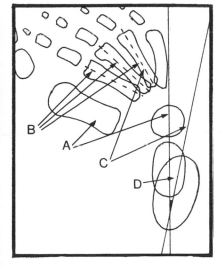

10. *Radiographs: A-P View:* (4) In club foot, the previously described relations are altered due to forefoot adduction. Note (A) talar axis does not cut the first met. (B) Middle met. axes are not parallel. (C) Calcaneal axis does not strike the fourth met. (D) Angle reduced.

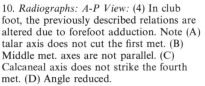

11. *Radiographs: Lateral:* (1) Draw (A) axes through talus and calcaneus, (B) tangents to the calcaneus and fifth metatarsal. Note (C) talar axis passes below the first metatarsal (at birth), (D) inter-axial angle is 25°–50°, (E) the angle between the tangents is 150°–175°.

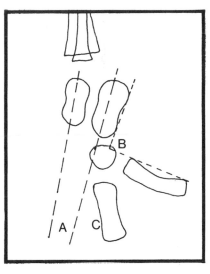

12. *Radiographs: Lateral:* (2) In club foot, note (A) talar and calcaneal axes nearly parallel, (B) the angle of the tangents is less obtuse, (C) the talar axis does not pass below the first metatarsal. Geometric analysis may be of help in the doubtful case and in assessing progress.

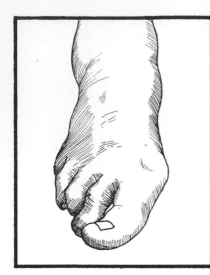

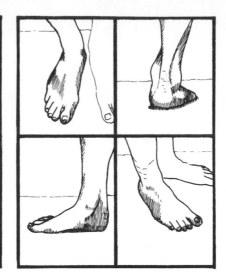

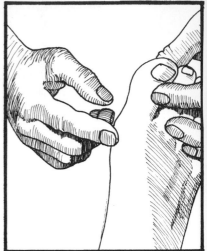

13. (1) *Appearance:* Note the shape of the foot, and the presence of any obvious deformities, abnormal callus formation, etc.

14. (2) *Weight-bearing posture:* Examine the weight-bearing foot, from above, from behind and from the sides.

15. (3) *Palpation:* Look for tenderness. Note any joint crepitations. Note any increase or decrease in skin temperature.

The mature foot — summary of key stages in examination (13–18)

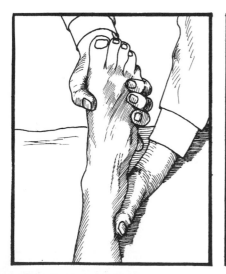

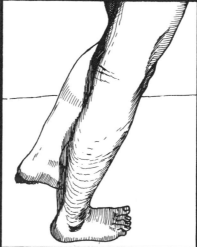

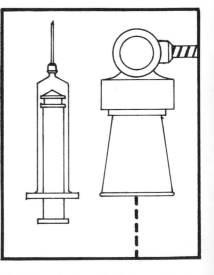

16. (4) *Movements:* Examine the mobility of the toes, foot and ankle.

17. (5) *Gait:* Examine the gait, with and without shoes. If indicated, screen the ankles, knees, hips, spine, CNS and the circulation. Note the footprint and examine the shoes.

18. (6) *Investigations:* Study the results of special investigations, e.g. radiographs, serum uric acid, sedimentation rate, Rose-Waaler test, etc.

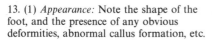

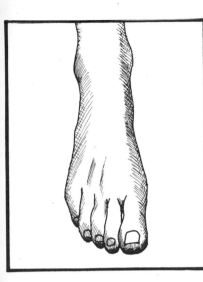

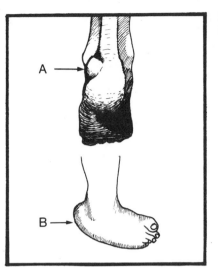

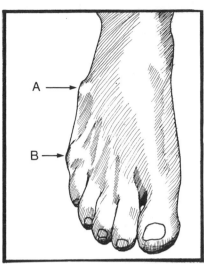

19. *Inspection: General:* Note if the foot is normally proportioned. If not, look at the hands and assess the rest of the skeleton. The feet for example are long and thin in Marfan's syndrome (arachnodactyly, spider bones).

20. *Inspection: Heel:* Is there (A) a calcaneal prominence ('calcaneal exostosis') with overlying callus or bursitis? Is there deformity of the heel suggesting old fracture or (B) talipes deformity?

21. *Inspection: Dorsum:* (1) Is there (A) prominence of the fifth metatarsal base? (B) An 'exostosis' from prominence of the fifth metatarsal head? (Both are sources of local pressure symptoms.)

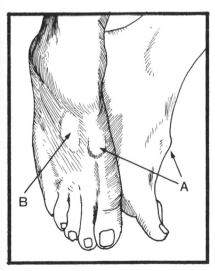

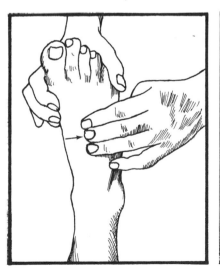

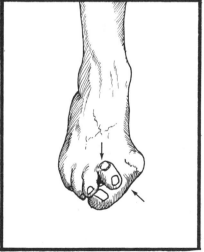

22. *Inspection: Dorsum:* (2) Is there (A) a cuneiform exostosis? (B) a dorsal ganglion?

23. *Inspection: Dorsum:* (3) Note the general state of the skin and nails. If there is any evidence of ischaemia, a full examination is required. In all cases, the presence of the dorsalis pedis pulse should be sought routinely.

24. *Inspection: Great toe:* (1) Note any hallux valgus deformity. If the deformity is severe, the great toe may under or over-ride the second, and it may pronate. The second toe may sublux at the M-P joint. Always re-assess any valgus deformity with the foot weight-bearing.

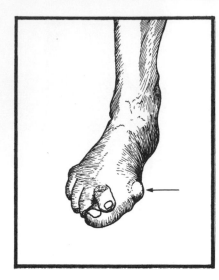

25. *Inspection: Great toe:* (2) Note the presence of any bursa over the M-P joint (bunion) and whether active inflammatory changes are present (from friction or infection). Discolouration of the joint with acute tenderness is suggestive of gout.

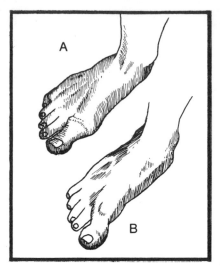

26. *Inspection: Great toe:* (3) Note if (A) the great toe is thickened at the M-P joint, suggesting hallux rigidus, or (B) held in a flexed position (hallux flexus).

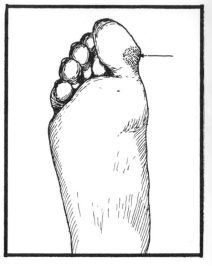

27. *Inspection: Great toe:* (4) Note the presence of excess callus under the great toe. This is suggestive of hallux rigidus.

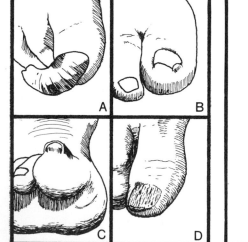

28. *Inspection: Great toe nail:* Note if the great toe nail is (A) deformed (onychogryphosis), (B) ingrowing, possibly with accompanying inflammation, (C) elevated (suggesting subungual exostosis), (D) of uneven texture and growth (suggesting fungal infection or psoriasis).

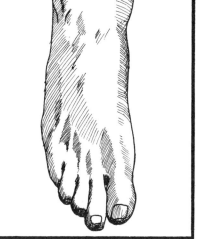

29. *Inspection: Toes:* (1) Note the relative lengths of the toes. A second toe longer than the first may occasionally become clawed or throw additional stresses on its M-P joint.

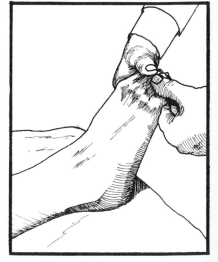

30. *Inspection: Toes:* (2) Flex the toes and note the relative lengths of the metatarsals. Abnormally short first or fifth metatarsals are a potential cause of forefoot imbalance and pain. When both are short, there is often painful callus under the second metatarsal.

THE FOOT 187

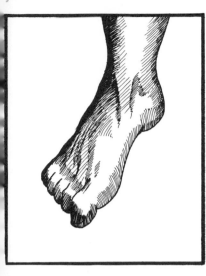

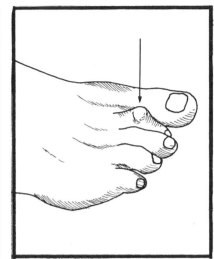

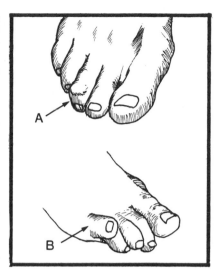

31. *Inspection: Toes:* (3) Claw toes. Are all the toes extended at the M-P joints and flexed at the I-P joints (claw toes), suggesting pes cavus or intrinsic muscle insufficiency?

32. *Inspection: Toes:* (4) Is there a hammer toe deformity (toe flexed at the proximal I-P joint)? The second toe is most commonly affected, often with an associated hallux valgus deformity. There is usually callus over the prominent I-P joint from shoe pressure.

33. *Inspection: Toes:* (5) Note the presence of (A) a mallet toe deformity (flexion deformity of the distal I-P joint). There is usually callus under the tip of the toe or deformity of the nail. (B) An overlapping fifth toe or quinti varus deformity (often congenital).

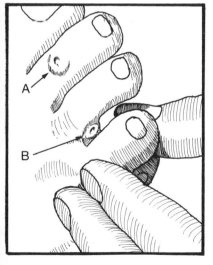

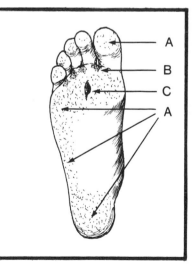

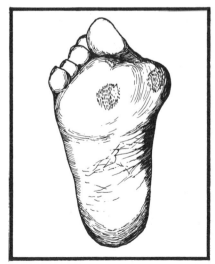

34. *Inspection: Toes:* (6) Note the presence of (A) hard corns. These are areas of hyperkeratosis which occur over bony prominences, generally through pressure against the shoes. (B) Soft corns are macerated hyperkeratotic lesions occurring between the toes.

35. *Inspection: Sole:* (1) Note (A) Hyperidrosis. (B) Evidence of fungal infection or athlete's foot. (C) Ulceration of sole suggesting pes cavus or neurological disturbance.

36. *Inspection: Sole:* (2) Note the presence of callus, indicating uneven or restricted area of weight-bearing. Be careful to distinguish between abnormal, local thickening, and *diffuse, moderate* thickening at the heel and under the metatarsal heads which is normal.

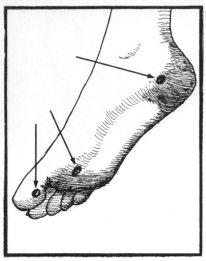

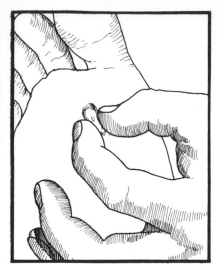

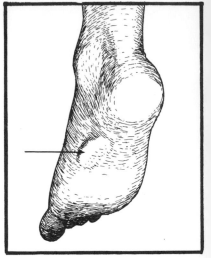

37. *Inspection: Sole:* (3) Note the presence of a verruca (plantar wart). Note the three classical sites. In the sole they are situated *between* the metatarsal heads: unlike callus, they do not occur in pressure areas.

38. *Verruca ctd.* A verucca is exquisitely sensitive to side to side pressure. Calluses are much less sensitive, and only to direct pressure. A magnifying lens may be used to confirm the central papillomatous structure of the verruca if there is any remaining doubt.

39. *Inspection: Sole:* (4) Note any localised fibrous tissue masses in the sole, arising from the plantar fascia and attached to the skin, occurring in Dupuytren's contracture of the feet. Always inspect the hands as both upper and lower limbs are often involved together.

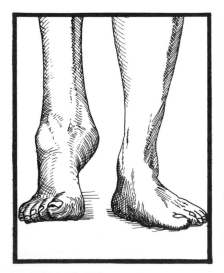

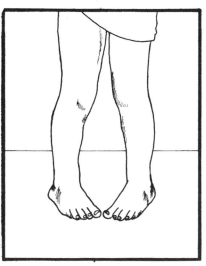

40. *Posture:* (1) Examine the patient standing. Are both the heel and forefoot squarely on the floor (plantigrade foot)? If the heel does not touch the ground, examine for shortening of the leg (see *Hip* 5) or shortening of the tendo-calcaneus (see *Ankle* 20).

41. *Posture:* (2) *Intoeing:* If this deformity is present, examine for (A) torsional deformity of the tibia (see *Tibia* 6), (B) increased internal rotation of the hips (see *Hip* 44), or (C) adduction of the forefoot. Most cases of intoeing in children resolve spontaneously by age 6.

42. *Posture:* (3) *Genu Valgum:* Note the presence of genu valgum which is frequently associated with valgus flat foot (see *Knee* 40).

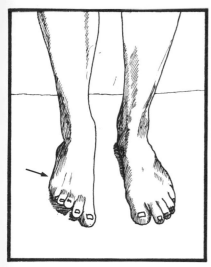

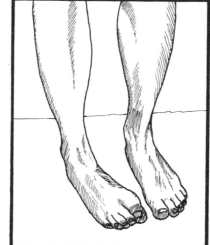

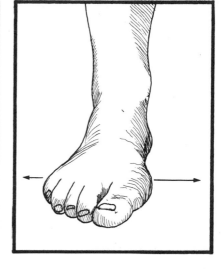

43. *Posture:* (4) *Eversion:* If the foot is everted, this suggests (A) peroneal spastic flat foot, (B) a painful lesion on the lateral side of the foot, (C) if less marked, pes planus.

44. *Posture:* (5) *Inversion:* If the foot is inverted, this suggests (A) muscle imbalance from stroke or other neurological disorder, (B) hallux flexus or rigidus, (C) pes cavus, (D) residual talipes deformity, (E) painful condition of the forefoot.

45. *Posture:* (6) *Splaying:* Note if there is broadening of the forefoot. This is often the result of intrinsic muscle weakness, and may be associated with pes cavus, callus under the metatarsal heads, hallux valgus, anterior metatarsalgia and trouble with shoe fitting.

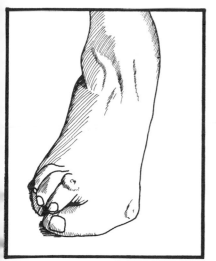

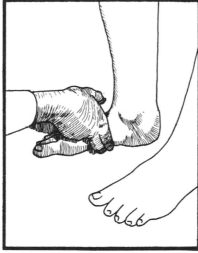

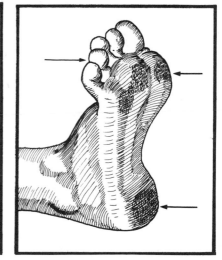

46. *Posture:* (7) *The toes:* Reassess the toes for clawing, mallet toes and hammer toes. Reassess the great toe, particularly for the degree of hallux valgus and over-riding of adjacent toe(s).

47. *Posture:* (8) *Medial Arch:* (1) Look at the arch and try to assess its height. Try to slip the fingers under the navicular. In *pes cavus*, the fingers may penetrate a distance of 2 cm or more from the vertical edge of the foot.

48. *Posture:* (9) *Medial Arch:* (2) If *pes cavus* is suggested, look for confirmatory clawing of the toes, callus or ulceration under the metatarsal heads, and alteration of the foot-print.

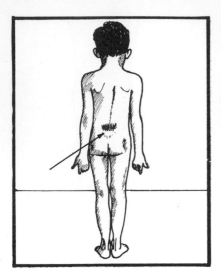

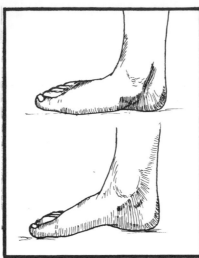

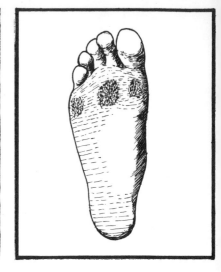

49. *Posture:* (10) *Medial Arch:* (3) If *pes cavus* is present, carry out a full neurological examination. Look at the lumbar spine for dimpling of the skin, a hairy patch, or pigmentation suggesting spina bifida or neurofififibromatosis. Radiography of the L/spine is desirable.

50. *Posture:* (11) *Medial Arch:* (4) In *pes planus*, the medial arch is obliterated. The navicular is often prominent, and the fingers cannot be inserted under it. Ask the patient to attempt to arch the foot. In mobile flat foot the arch can often be restored voluntarily.

51. *Posture:* (12) *Medial Arch:* (5) If *pes planus* is suspected, re-examine the sole for evidence of an increase in the area of weight-bearing. The footprint will be abnormal in these circumstances. Note also the presence of knock-knee deformity (see *Knee* 40).

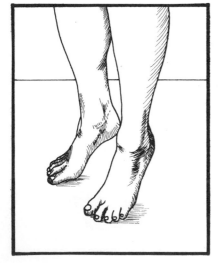

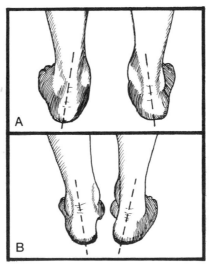

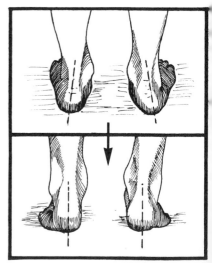

52. *Posture:* (13) *Medial Arch:* (6) Pes planus. Assess the mobility of the foot first by asking the patient to stand on the toes, at the same time examining the alteration in the shape of the foot by sight and feel. Later in examination carefully note inversion and eversion range.

53. *Posture:* (14) *Heel:* (1) Look at the foot from behind, paying particular attention to the slope of the heels. Note (A) valgus heels are associated with pes planus. (B) Varus heels are associated with pes cavus.

54. *Posture:* (15) *Heel:* (2) Again ask the patient to stand on the toes, observing the heels. If the heel posture corrects, this indicates a mobile sub-talar joint. Where the heel is valgus it may suggest shortening of the tendo calcaneus.

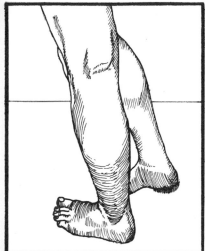

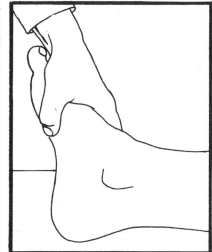

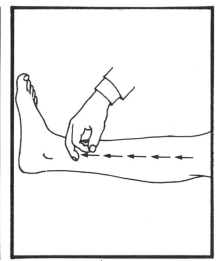

55. *Gait:* Watch the patient walking, first bare-footed and then in shoes, to assess the gait. Examine from behind, from in front, and from the side. A child should also be made to run. A reluctant child can usually be coaxed to walk holding its mother's hand.

56. *Skin temperature:* Grasp the foot and assess the skin temperature, comparing one side with the other. Take into account the effects of local bandaging and the ambient temperature. A warm foot is particularly suggestive of rheumatoid arthritis or gout.

57. *Circulation:* (1) If the foot is cold, note the skin temperature gradient along the length of the limb. You should have already observed any trophic changes or discolouration of the skin suggestive of ischaemia.

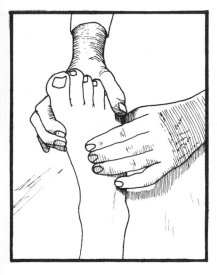

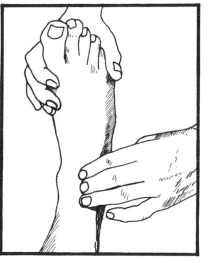

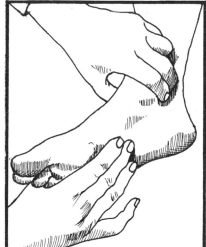

58. *Circulation:* (2) Attempt to palpate the dorsalis pedis artery. The vessel lies just lateral to the tendon of extensor hallucis longus and its pulsation should be felt against the middle cuneiform. A good pulse is against any significant degree of ischaemia.

59. *Circulation:* (3) Now try to feel the anterior tibial pulse near the midline of the ankle just above the joint line, where the vessel crosses the distal end of the tibia.

60. *Circulation:* (4) The posterior tibial artery is often difficult to find, and it is helpful to invert the foot while palpating behind the medial malleolus.

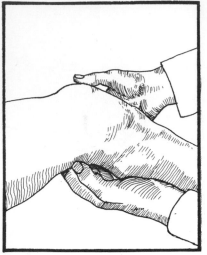

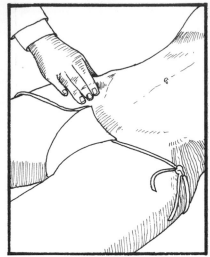

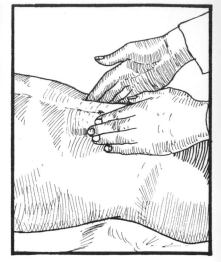

61. *Circulation:* (5) Next seek the popliteal artery. When the patient is supine it can only be felt by applying strong pressure in an anterior direction, with the knee flexed, to force the vessel against the femoral condyles. Alternatively it may be sought with the patient prone.

62. *Circulation:* (6) The femoral pulse may be felt a little to the medial side of the mid-point of the groin, when the artery can be compressed against the superior pubic ramus.

63. *Circulation:* (7) Examine the abdomen, palpating the abdominal aorta. Note the presence of pulsation as it is compressed against the lumbar spine, and note any evidence of aneurysmal dilatation.

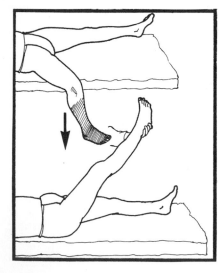

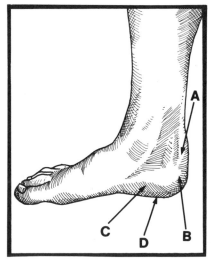

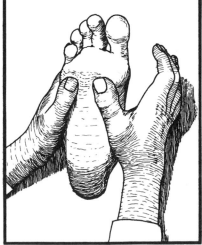

64. *Circulation:* (8) Note any cyanosis of the foot when dependent and blanching on elevation suggestive of marked arterial insufficiency.

65. *Tenderness:* (1) *Heel:* Tenderness round the heel is present in
(A) Sever's disease.
(B) Calcaneal exostosis, tendo calcaneus bursitis.
(C) Plantar fasciitis.
(D) Pes cavus.

66. *Tenderness:* (2) *Forefoot:* (1) Diffuse tenderness under all the metatarsal heads is common in
(A) Anterior metatarsalgia.
(B) Pes cavus and pes planus.
(C) Gout and rheumatoid arthritis.

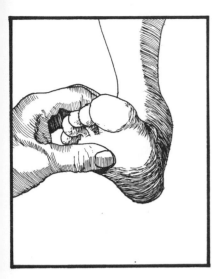

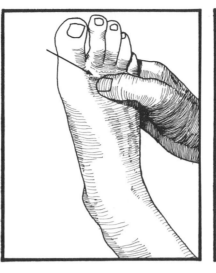

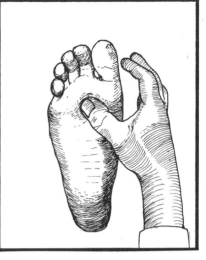

67. *Tenderness:* (3) *Forefoot:* (2) Tenderness under the second metatarsal head and over the metatarso-phalangeal joint is found when the second toe subluxes as a sequel to hallux valgus or rheumatoid arthritis.

68. *Tenderness:* (4) *Forefoot:* (3) Puffy, localised swelling on the dorsum of the foot, palpable thickening of the second M-P joint, pain on plantar-flexion of the toe, and joint tenderness are diagnostic of *Freiberg's disease.*

69. *Tenderness* (5) *Forefoot:* (4) Tenderness on *both* plantar and dorsal surface of the second or third metatarsal necks or shafts occurs in March fracture.

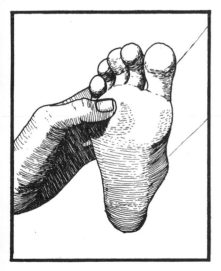

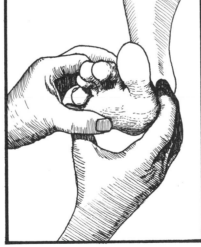

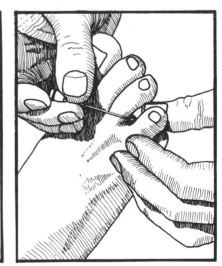

70. *Tenderness:* (6) *Forefoot:* (5) *Plantar neuroma:* Sharply defined tenderness between the metatarsal heads (most commonly between the third and fourth) is found in *plantar digital neuroma.*

71. *Plantar neuroma:* (2) *Morton's metatarsalgia:* Occasionally the neuroma may be felt to move by compressing the metatarsal heads with one hand while simultaneously pressing from the sole towards the dorsal surface and back.

72. *Plantar neuroma:* (3) Sometimes the patient complains of paraesthesiae in the toes, and sensory impairment should be sought on both sides of the web space involved.

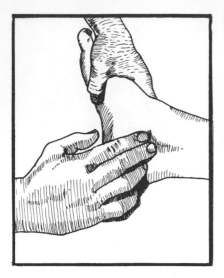

73. *Tenderness:* (7) *Tarsal tunnel syndrome:* (1) Tenderness may occur over the posterior tibial nerve in the tarsal tunnel syndrome.

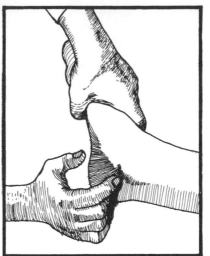

74. *Tarsal tunnel syndrome:* (2) Tapping over the posterior tibial nerve may give rise to paraesthesiae in the foot in this condition.

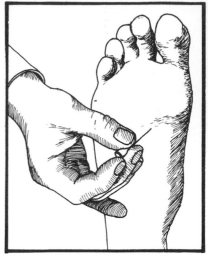

75. *Tarsal tunnel syndrome:* (3) Test sensation over the whole of the sole of the foot and the toes in the area of supply of the medial and lateral plantar nerves (the two terminal divisions of the posterior tibial nerve). Compare the feet (loss is rather uncommon).

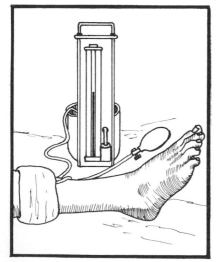

76. *Tarsal tunnel syndrome:* (4) In doubtful cases, apply a tourniquet to the calf and inflate to just above the systolic blood pressure. If this brings on the patient's symptoms in 1–2 minutes, the diagnosis is confirmed.

77. *Tenderness:* (8) *Great toe:* (1) *In gout,* tenderness is often most acute, but is diffusely spread round the whole M-P joint and often the entire toe. There is often bluish discolouration of the skin round the toe.

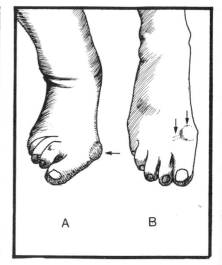

78. *Tenderness:* (9) *Great toe:* (2)
(A) *In hallux valgus* tenderness is often absent or confined to the bunion.
(B) *In hallux rigidus* there is tenderness over the exostoses which form on the metatarsal head and proximal phalanx, often on the dorsal surface as well.

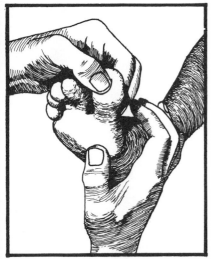

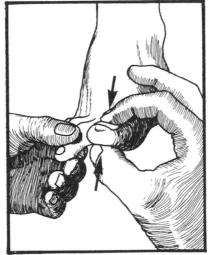

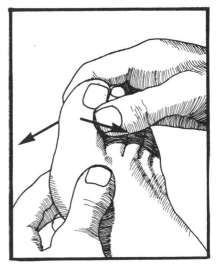

79. *Tenderness:* (10) *In sesamoiditis,* there is tenderness over the sesamoid bones which are situated under the first metatarsal head. Pain is produced if the toe is dorsiflexed while pressure is maintained on the sesamoid bones.

80. *Tenderness:* (11) *Great toe nail:* In subungual exostosis, pain is produced by squeezing the toe in the vertical plane. In ingrowing toe nail, pain is produced by side to side pressure.

81. *Crepitations:* Move the toe in an up and down direction while palpating the M-P joint. Repeat with the I-P joint. Crepitations, indicating O-A changes are constant in the M-P joint in hallux rigidus. I-P creps are a contraindication for M-P joint fusion.

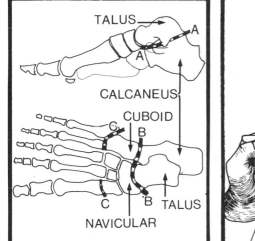

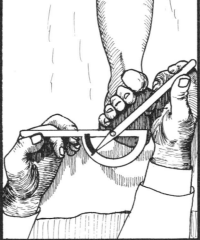

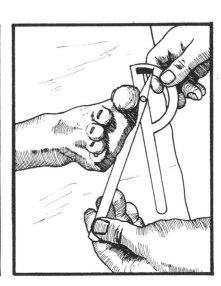

82. *Movements:* (1) Note that in the normal foot (A) 80% of inversion/eversion is mediated through the sub-talar joint; the calcaneus rolls, pitches and yaws under the talus, carrying the rest of the foot with it. (B) Most of the remainder occurs at the mid-tarsal joint. (C) A little takes place at the tarso-metatarsal joints, particularly at the first, fourth and fifth.

83. *Movements:* (1) *Inversion:* Ask the patient to turn the soles of the feet towards one another. The patellae should be vertical. The resulting angle may be measured. If the legs are squarely placed on the couch its end may be used as a guide.
Normal range = 35° approx.

84. *Movements:* (2) *Eversion:* Ask the patient to turn the feet outwards. The range of movement may be measured in a similar fashion.
Normal range = 20° approx.

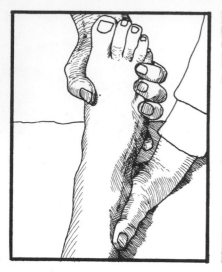

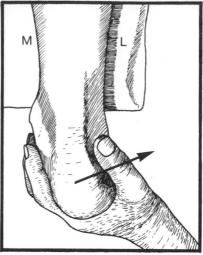

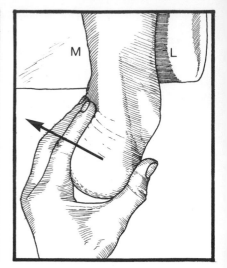

85. *Movements:* (3) If inversion and eversion are restricted, fix the heel with one hand and assist the patient with the other to repeat the movements. No reduction in the range = a stiff subtalar joint. Presence of some movement shows that the mid-tarsa and tarso-metatarsal joints preserve some mobility.

86. *Movements:* (4) Turn the patient face down with the feet over the edge of the examination couch. Evert the heel and note the presence of movement in the sub-talar joint by the position of the heel. The normal range of eversion of the heel is about 10°.

87. *Movements:* (5) Repeat, forcing the heel into inversion. The normal range of inversion measurable at the heel is about 20°. Loss of movements indicates a stiff sub-talar joint (e.g. old calcaneal fracture, rheumatoid or osteo-arthritis, spastic flat foot.

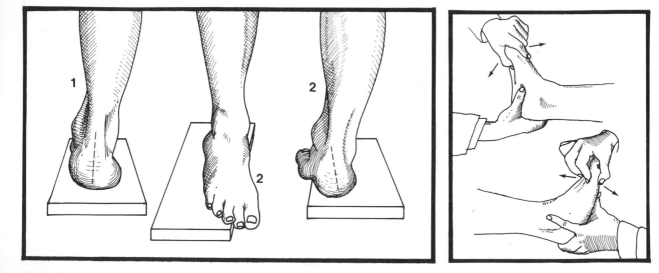

88. *Movements:* (6) In idiopathic pes cavus, and pes cavus secondary to neuromuscular disease, the sub-talar joint is generally mobile; in pes cavus secondary to congenital talipes equinovarus the sub-talar joint is often stiff. As a further guide to the differentiation of these cases, mark the axis of the heel with a skin pencil, and note its position with the patient standing on a 2 cm block of wood — first squarely (1), and then with the forefoot over the medial edge (2). A change in the axis (3) indicates a mobile sub-talar joint.

89. *Movements:* (7) Test for mobility in the first, fourth and fifth tarso-metatarsal joints by steadying the heel with one hand and attempting to move the metatarsal heads individually in a dorsal and plantar direction.

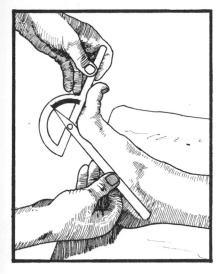

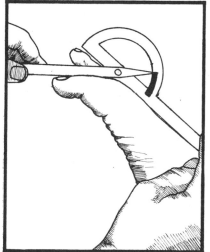

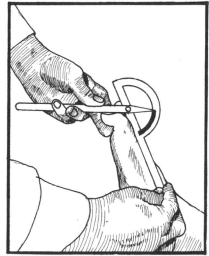

90. *Movements:* (8) *Great toe:* Note the range of extension in the great toe at the M-P joint.
Normal range = 65°

91. *Movements:* (9) *Great toe:* Note the range of flexion at the M-P joint. *Normal range* = 40°. M-P movements are severely restricted and painful in hallux rigidus. There is often little impairment in hallux valgus unless secondary arthritic changes are quite severe.

92. *Movements:* (10) *Great toe:* Note the range in the I-P joint. *Normal flexion* = 60°. *Extension* = 0°. Restriction is common after fractures of the terminal phalanx, and is a contraindication to M-P joint fusion.

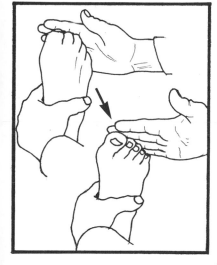

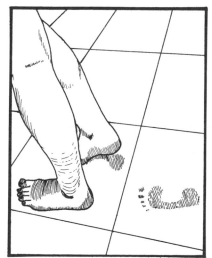

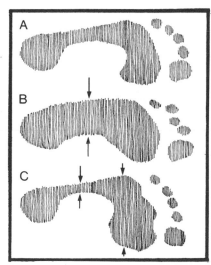

93. *Movements:* (11) *Toes:* Overall mobility may be roughly assessed by alternately curling and straightening the toes. Accurate measurement of individual ranges is seldom needed. Restriction is often seen in gout, rheumatoid arthritis, Sudeck's atrophy and ischaemic conditions of the foot and leg.

94. *Footprint:* (1) It is sometimes helpful to see the pattern of weight distribution in the foot. Note the imprint of the sweaty foot on a vinyl floor, or (A) apply olive oil to the sole and dust the imprint with talc, (B) use ink on paper (or 'fix' on an X-ray plate and develop it). A pedoscope may also be used for this purpose.

95. *Footprint:* (2) *Typical patterns:* (A) Normal foot. (B) Pes planus. Note increase in area of central part of sole taking part in weight-bearing. (C) Pes cavus. Note decrease in area of contact in mid-sole and anterior splaying. In extreme cases the lateral weight-bearing strip may disappear.

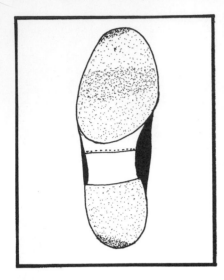

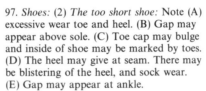

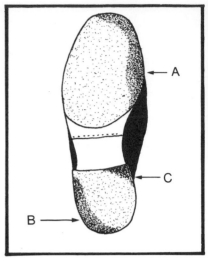

96. *Shoes:* (1) The patient's only complaint may be shoe wear. Inspection is expected and may be helpful. In the normal sole wear is fairly even, being maximal across the tread and at the tip (to the lateral side). At the back of the heel, maximum wear is also to the lateral side.

97. *Shoes:* (2) *The too short shoe:* Note (A) excessive wear toe and heel. (B) Gap may appear above sole. (C) Toe cap may bulge and inside of shoe may be marked by toes. (D) The heel may give at seam. There may be blistering of the heel, and sock wear. (E) Gap may appear at ankle.

98. *Shoes* (3) *Pes planus:* (1)
(A) Wear on medial side of sole extending to the tip.
(B) Wear on outer side of heel.
(C) In severe cases, wear on diagonal corner of heel.

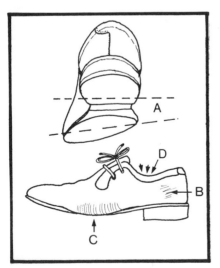

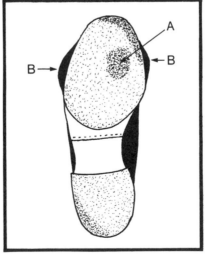

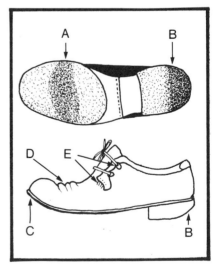

99. *Shoes:* (4) *Pes planus:* (2)
(A) Shoe twisted when viewed from behind (heel and sole on different planes).
(B) Scuff marks on medial side.
(C) The upper bulges over the sole on the medial side.
(D) The quarter bulges away from the foot.

100. *Shoes:* (5) *Splay foot:* (3) Note
(A) Excess wear in the region of the first or second metatarsal heads.
(B) The upper bulges over the sole anteriorly.

101. *Shoes:* (6) *Pes cavus:* Note
(A) Excessive wear under the metatarsal head region.
(B) Excessive wear at back of heel.
(C) Raising of toe.
(D) Creases.
(E) Giving way of lacings.

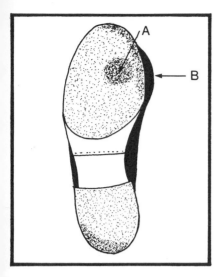

102. *Shoes:* (7) *Hallux valgus:* There is often (A) excess wear as in splay foot under the area of the first and second metatarsal heads; (B) bulging of upper to accommodate the prominent first metatarsal head.

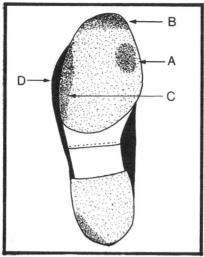

103. *Shoes:* (8) *Hallux rigidus:* Note (A) excessive wear under the first metatarsal head and (B) at the tip of the sole. (C) Excess wear on the lateral side (through walking on the side of the foot). (D) Lateral overhang. The toe of the shoe may be up-turned.

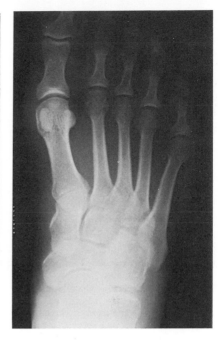

104. *Radiographs:* (1) Normal A-P radiograph of the foot.

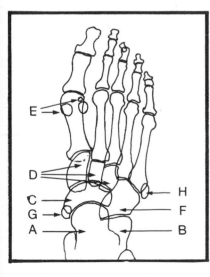

105. *Radiographs:* (2) An A-P is routine, with a lateral or oblique. (A) Talus. (B) Calcaneus. (C) Navicular. (D) Cuneiforms. (E) Sesamoids (often bi- or tri-partite). (F) Cuboid. Inconstant accessory bones may be mistaken for fracture or loose bodies, e.g. (G) os tibiale externum. (H) Os vesalianum.

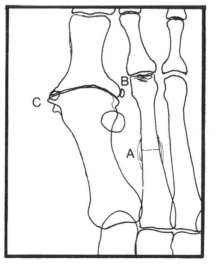

106. *Radiographs:* (3) in the A-P view, note bone texture and typical anomalies such as (A) March fracture (periosteal reaction occurs in healing stages), (B) Freiberg's disease, (C) O-A changes with exostosis formation (hallux rigidus).

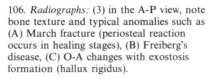

107. *Radiographs:* (4) Note, if present, (A) metatarsus primus varus. (B) First metatarsal 'exostosis'. (C) Hallux valgus. (D) Joint narrowing or cyst formation suggestive of O-A, R-A or gout. (E) M-P joint subluxation secondary to hallux valgus or to rheumatoid arthritis.

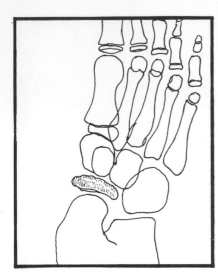

108. *Radiographs:* (5) In the child note any increased density of the navicular suggestive of Kohler's disease. The bone may appear reduced in size.

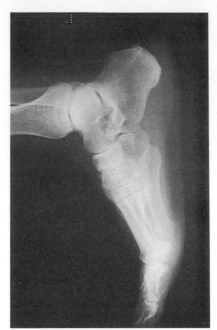

109. *Radiographs:* (6) Normal lateral radiograph of the foot.

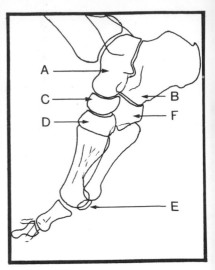

110. *Radiographs:* (7) In the lateral radiograph, it is often difficult to trace the outline of individual metatarsals due to superimposition, although the first and fifth are usually quite clear. (A) Talus, (B) calcaneus, (C) navicular, (D) med. cuneiform, (E) sesamoid, (F) cuboid.

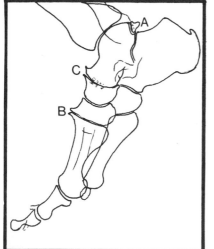

111. *Radiographs:* (8) Note if present (A) the accessory os trigonum (often mistaken for a fracture), (B) cuneiform exostosis, (C) narrowing of the mid-tarsal joint and other changes suggestive of mid-tarsal rheumatoid or osteo-arthritis.

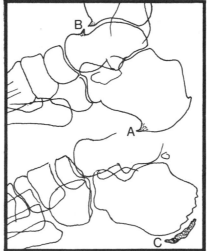

112. *Radiographs:* (9) Note if present in the adult (A) calcaneal spur, sometimes associated with plantar fasciitis, (B) footballer's ankle, (C) in the child, increased density and fragmentation of the calcaneal epiphysis, seen in Sever's disease.

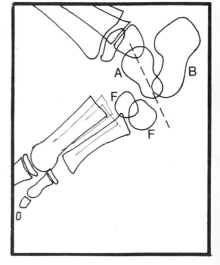

113. *Radiographs:* (10) Congenital vertical talus which is associated with dislocation of the talo-navicular joint has a classical radiographic appearance. Note the direction of the long axis of the talus. (A) Talus, (B) calcaneus, (F) both centres of ossification in the cuboid.

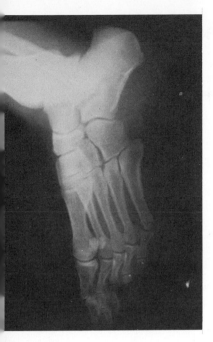

114. *Radiographs:* (11) Normal oblique radiograph of the foot.

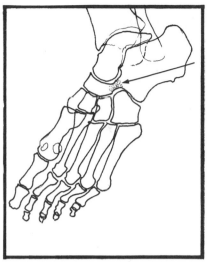

115. *Radiographs:* (12) Calcaneo-navicular bar or synostosis is best seen in oblique projections of the foot, and is found in association with spastic flat foot.

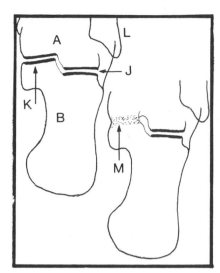

116. *Radiographs:* (13) An axial or tangential projection of the heel shows (A) talus, (B) calcaneus, (J) posterior talo-calcaneal joint, (K) sustentaculum tali, (L) base of fifth metatarsal. A talo-calcaneal synostosis, sometimes found in spastic flat foot, may be demonstrated by this view (M).

117. *Radiographs:* (14) A tangential projection may be used when the sesamoid bones are suspect, showing for example (A) osteo-chondritic changes, (B) stress fracture.

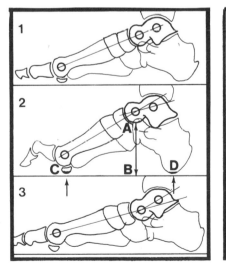

118. *Radiographs:* (15) A weight-bearing lateral projection is of value in assessing deformities involving the longitudinal arches and toes. The axes of the talus and first metatarsal normally coincide, and the height of the arch may be assessed by noting the ratio AB/CD. (1) Normal, (2) pes cavus, (3) pes planus.

119. *Radiographs:* (16) In the assessment of hallux valgus, the A-P projection should always be taken weight-bearing. Note how a reference line through the second metatarsal is used when taking measurements, (A) primus varus deformity of 20°, (B) hallux valgus deformity of 35°.

Biochemical Values

	Serum calcium	Serum phosphate	Alkaline phosphatase	Total acid phosphatase	Remarks
Normal range	2.12–2.62 mmol/litre 8.5–10.5 mg/100 cc	Adults: 0.8–1.4 mmol/litre 2.5–4.3 mg/100 cc; Children: 1.3–2.0 mmol/litre 4–6.2 mg/100 cc	Adults: 21–106; Children: 21–142; Infants: 21–210 IU/litre	2.0–5.5 IU/litre	
Laboratory accuracy	±2%	±2%	±10%	±10%	
Hyper-parathyroidism	Raised	Lowered	Raised if bone involved	Normal	
Hypo-parathyroidism	Lowered	Raised	Normal	Normal	
Pseudo hypo-parathyroidism	Lowered	Raised	Normal	Normal	
Osteoporosis	Normal	Normal	Normal	Normal	
Osteomalacia	Normal to low	Low	Slight increase	Normal	Ca X PO$_4$ < 2.25 SI units or 28.0 mg/100 cc units
Rickets	Normal to low	Low	Slight increase	Normal	
Paget's disease	Normal, raised in immobilisation	Normal	Raised	Raised	
Uraemic osteodystrophy	Low or normal	Raised	Raised	Normal	
Myelomatosis	Often raised	Normal	Normal	Normal	High ESR
Bone metastases	Normal or raised	Normal or low	Raised	Normal or raised	ESR raised
Sarcoidosis	Often raised	Usually normal	Normal	Normal	ESR raised
Prostatic neoplasm	Normal or raised	Normal or low	Normal or high	Normal or high raised in 15% of cases without and in 65% with metastases	Prostatic acid phosphatase fraction of total acid phosphatase affected but not in highly malignant undifferentiated tumours

	SI units	*mg/100 cc or ug/100 cc*
Total serum protein	60–80 g/litre	6.0–8.0 mg/100 cc
Albumin	33–50 g/litre	3.3–5.0 mg/100 cc
Globulin	20–35 g/litre	2.0–3.5 mg/100 cc
Bilirubin	5–20 μmol/litre	0.29–1.17 mg/100 cc
Urea	2.5–7.5 mmol/litre	15–45 mg/100 cc
Serum urate	Males: 0.13–0.45 mmol/litre	2.2–7.6 mg/100 cc
	Females: 0.13–0.35 mmol/litre	2.2–5.9 mg/100 cc
Serum iron	Males: 14–32 μmol/litre	78–180 μg/100 cc
	Females: 10–30 μmol/litre	56–168 μg/100 cc
Total iron binding capacity (TIBC)	45–70 μmol/litre	250–390 μg/100 cc
Fasting blood Glucose	3.3–5.6 mmol/litre	60–100 mg/100 cc
Serum cholesterol	3.6–8.5 mmol/litre	140–330 mg/100 cc

Radiographic Section

The following section is intended as an exercise in the interpretation of significant points in the history, important clinical findings, and relevant radiographs of a series of cases. These have been arranged in the same order as the first sections of the book, starting with the cervical spine.

The answers to these problems in diagnosis are given in numerical order in the pages following the radiographs. Cross references, unless otherwise stated, refer to caption numbers in the corresponding clinical sections.

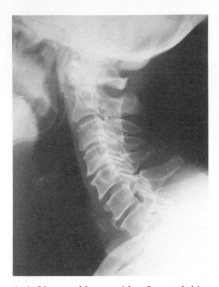

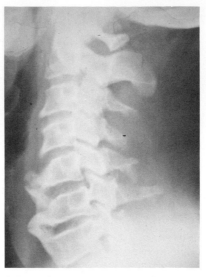

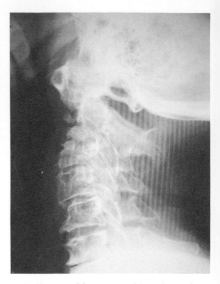

1. A 56 year old man with a five week history of pain in the neck radiating into the right shoulder: clinically, there was moderate restriction of all neck movements, with pain at the extremes of rotation. No abnormal neurological signs were found.

2. Lateral cervical radiograph of a 72 year old man with a six week history of dysphagia. On clinical examination he was found to have gross restriction of all cervical movements.

3. A 68 year old woman with a six week history of increasing weakness of the arms and legs: she had suffered from rheumatoid arthritis for many years. Weakness involving the main muscle groups in all four limbs was confirmed, and the plantar reflexes were extensor.

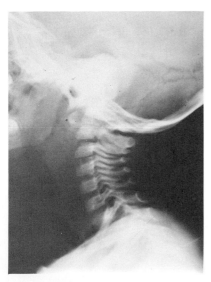

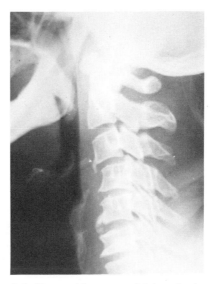

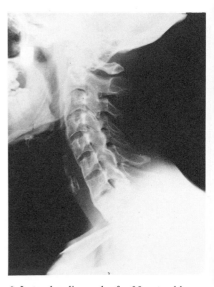

4. Lateral radiograph of a four year old child with a three month history of malaise, weight loss and neck pain particularly troublesome at night. The child supported his head with his hands, and resented any attempt at examination of the neck.

5. A 65 year old man complaining of pain in the neck following a fall down stairs four days previously. There was a past history of recurrent neck pain. Clinically there was marked restriction of all neck movements, and an occipital haematoma. No neurological abnormality noted.

6. Lateral radiograph of a 35 year old man with a two year history of progressive stiffness of the neck and back, associated with fleeting back pain. The sedimentation rate was 87mm in the first hour, and the Rose-Waaler test negative. Marked spinal stiffness was confirmed.

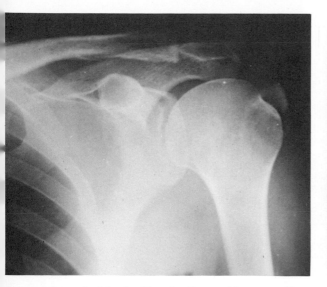

7. A-P radiograph of the shoulder of a 41 year old woman with a three day history of acute pain in the shoulder. She supported the affected arm with the other, and would not permit any movement of the affected joint. The shoulder was warm to touch and there was marked widespread tenderness. The white blood count and sedimentation rate were normal.

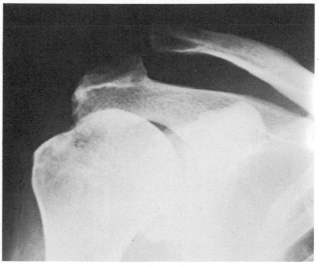

8. Radiograph of the right shoulder, taken in the erect position, of a 22 year old man complaining of unilateral shoulder pain one week after a road traffic accident. A previous radiograph had been reported as showing no abnormality. On clinical examination there was some prominence and local tenderness over the lateral extremity of the clavicle.

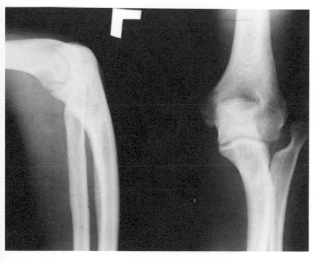

9. A 42 year old housewife complained of progressive weakness and paraesthesiae in the left hand. She was found to have a partial ulnar nerve palsy. She was noted to have a cubitus varus deformity, with a bony prominence over the lateral aspect of the joint. There was some tenderness along the line of the ulnar nerve which was thickened. The patient gave a history of an injury to the elbow in childhood.

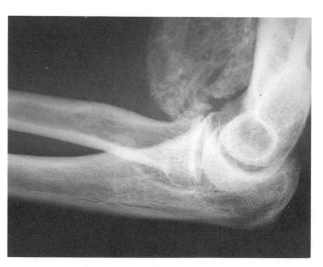

10. Lateral radiograph of the elbow of a 30 year old man who had sustained a severe head injury four months previously. No injury to the joint had been recorded at the time of his admission, but he was later found to have gross restriction of flexion in the elbow.

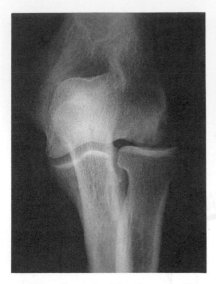

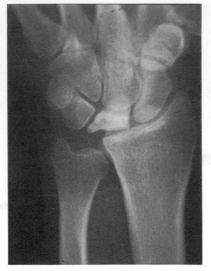

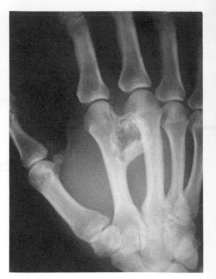

11. A-P radiograph of the elbow of a 22 year old man with a six month history of aching pain in the elbow. Clinical examination revealed pain at the extremes of pronation and supination, but little else in the way of positive findings.

12. Radiograph of the wrist of a 24 year old woman with a nine month history of pain and swelling of the joint. There was slight puffy swelling on the dorsum of the wrist, proximal carpal tenderness, and limitation of movements.

13. Oblique radiograph of the hand of a 28 year old man who had been aware for many months of a painless swelling near the knuckle of the index metacarpal. An isolated, hard swelling arising from bone was confirmed at this site.

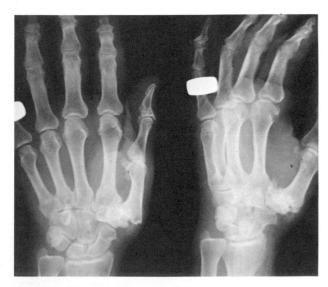

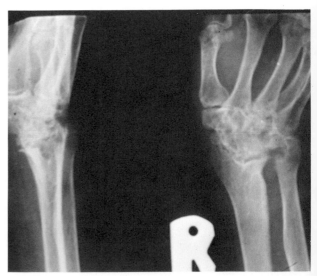

14. A-P and oblique radiographs of the hand of a 65 year old man complaining of increasing pain at the base of the thumb over the previous year. He also complained of weakness of grip. On clinical examination marked prominence of the thumb metacarpal was observed. Crepitations were noted at the base of the thumb on both active and passive movements.

15. Radiographs of a 22 year old woman complaining of pain, swelling, stiffness and weakness of the right wrist, becoming progressively worse over the last nine months. She was noted to have marked swelling of the wrist, with muscle wasting in the hand and forearm. All wrist movements were found to be seriously impaired and painful. No other joints were involved. The Rose-Waaler test was negative.

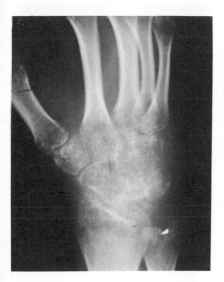

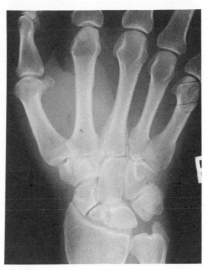

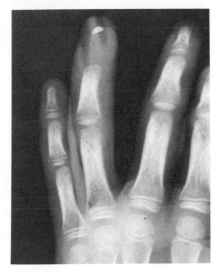

16. A 55 year old woman complained of pain and swelling of the hand and fingers 3 weeks after plaster fixation for a minor wrist injury had been discarded. The fingers and hand were swollen, all movements of the fingers grossly restricted, and the wrist diffusely tender.

17. A 35 year old man complained of pain and stiffness over the last year in the right wrist. A history was obtained of a wrist injury 6 years previously. He was found to have slight limitation of all wrist movements except pronation/supination.

18. A 10 year old boy had a three week history of a septic finger following a puncture wound of the ring finger. On clinical examination the whole finger was rather swollen, and there was a purulent discharge from the pulp.

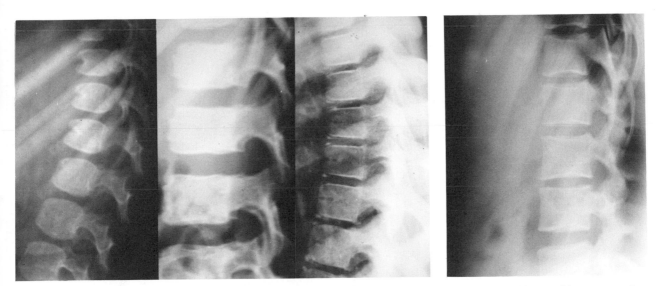

19. The three radiographs above are of patients who were being investigated for backache. *In the first*, note the indented appearance of the upper three vertebral bodies. *In the second*, note the projections from the anterior margins of the vertebral bodies. *In the third*, observe the patchy cystic shadows in the vertebral bodies and the dense opacities present between the bodies anteriorly.

20. A 20 year old man with a two month history of upper lumbar pain; there was no history of trauma. Clinically, movements in the lumbar spine were restricted, and there was tenderness and muscle spasm. No abnormal neurological signs were detected. The ESR was 43 mm.

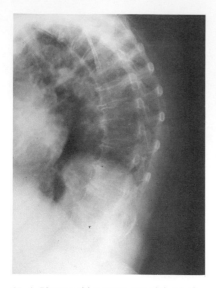

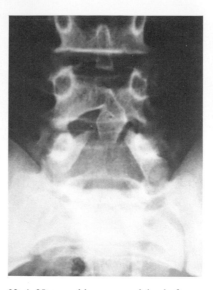

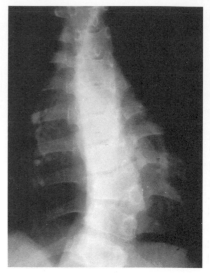

21. A 78 year old woman complained of dorsal backache over several years. She was noted to have a marked regular dorsal kyphosis, with almost complete loss of movements in the dorsal spine. The serum calcium and phosphate were within normal limits.

22. A 28 year old man complained of increasing pain under the metatarsal heads of both feet. He was found to have severe bilateral pes cavus. Radiographic examination of the spine was carried out, although no neurological abnormality was noted in the lower limbs.

23. A-P radiograph of a 12 year old boy who, although symptom free, had been brought for examination by his mother who was concerned about the shape of his back. Clinically he was found to have a fixed (structural) scoliosis.

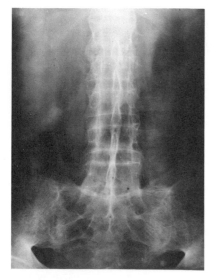

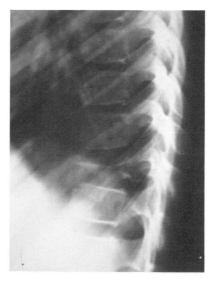

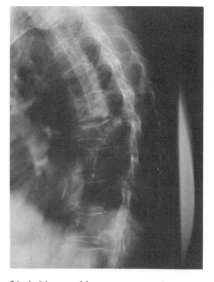

24. A 35 year old man complained of diffuse, intermittent back pain over several years, with increasing spinal stiffness. He was found to have a regular dorsal kyphosis, gross restriction of spinal movements, pulmonary tuberculosis and a sedimentation rate of 95 mm in one hour.

25. Lateral radiograph of a girl of ten who gave a 6 week history of lower thoracic spinal pain. On clinical examination she was found to have a slight angular kyphosis, pain on forward flexion, and a raised sedimentation rate. The diagnosis was confirmed by biopsy.

26. A 64 year old woman gave a 3 month history of back pain, with no history of trauma. The spine of D9 was prominent and tender. There was slight, painful restriction of thoracic spinal movements. The ESR was 12 mm, and the serum calcium and phosphate were 2.14 and 0.79.

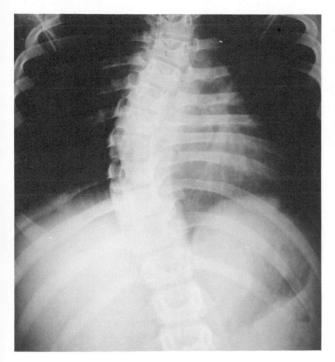

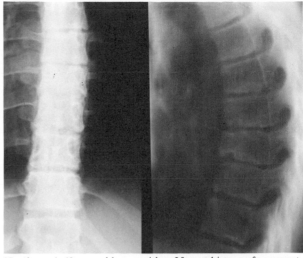

27. *Above:* A 40 year old man with a 25 year history of recurrent thoracic spinal pain. He had a marked, regular dorsal kyphosis, with little movement detectable in the dorsal spine. 28. *Left:* A-P radiograph of the dorsal spine of a 13 year old girl who was noted to have a scoliotic deformity. On clinical examination she was found to have a fixed thoracic curve convex to the right, and rib-cage deformity.

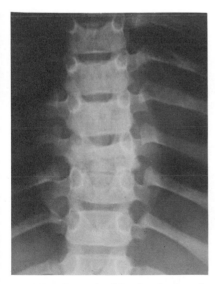

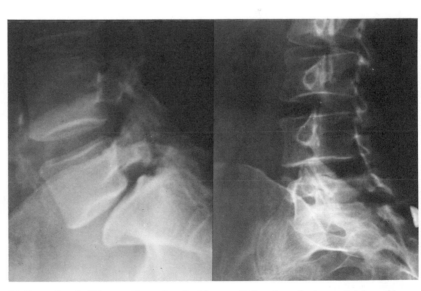

29. A-P radiograph of the dorsal spine of an 8 year old boy with a 3 month history of general malaise, back pain, and night sweats. There was marked restriction of spinal movements, with much protective spasm. There was pain on percussion of the thoracic spine.

30. Lateral and oblique radiographs of a 38 year old female patient complaining of low back pain radiating into both buttocks. Symptoms had been present with various degrees of severity for several years. She stood with an increased lumbar lordosis, and the first piece of the sacrum was unduly prominent. No abnormal neurological signs were elicited in the lower limbs.

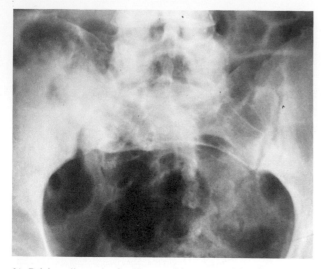

31. Pelvic radiograph of a 25 year old woman with a five week history of pain to the right of the sacrum. There was general malaise and pyrexia. Some fullness and marked tenderness were noted over the right sacro-iliac joint. Attempts to spring the joint gave rise to great pain. The white blood count and sedimentation rate were both raised.

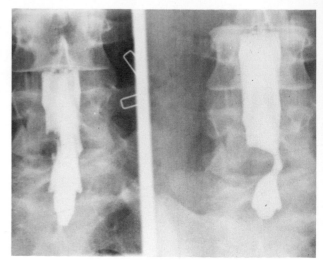

32. Myelogram performed on a 27 year old man with a six month history of backache and right sided sciatic pain. He had been treated by bed rest and analgesics without improvement. There was loss of lumbar lordosis and restriction of flexion. Straight leg raising was positive on the right at 30°. There was weakness of dorsiflexion and eversion, and some sensory impairment over the lateral aspect of the right calf.

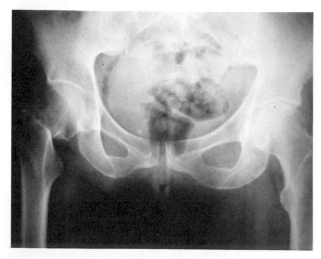

33. Pelvic radiograph of a 70 year old woman with a week's history of pain in the right groin and inability to weight bear. A history of a minor fall prior to the onset of the symptoms was obtained. Some external rotation deformity of the right hip was noted, and there was true shortening of the leg amounting to 2 cm. Pain was elicited at the extremes of movement of the right hip.

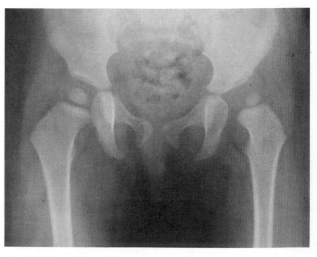

34. A-P view of the pelvis to show both hips of a 17 month old girl who had been noted to be walking with a painless limp. Clinical examination suggested some shortening of the left leg, and there was restriction of abduction at 90° flexion.

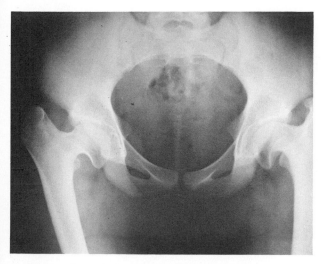

35. Pelvic radiograph of a 25 year old woman who was complaining of aching pain in both hips. She was of small stature and walked with a waddling gait. There was moderate restriction of all movements in both hips, although abduction was particularly affected.

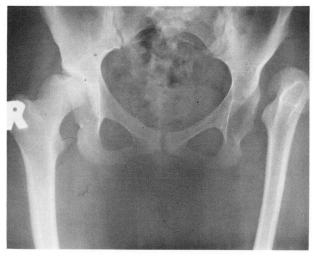

36. Pelvic radiograph of a 20 year old girl complaining of increasing pain over the last two years in the right hip. She gave a history of a painless limp affecting the other hip from childhood. On clinical examination she was noted to have an increased lumbar lordosis. The left hip was prominent and there was shortening of the left leg. Rotation of the right hip was slightly restricted and painful.

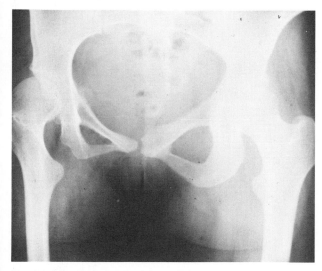

37. This pelvic radiograph is of an adult patient who gave a history of poliomyelitis affecting her right leg in childhood. Three characteristic confirmatory deformities were observed on the film.

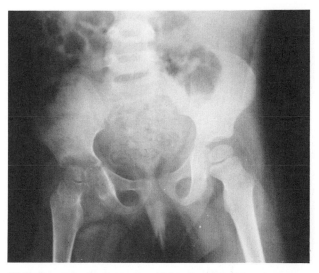

38. Radiograph of a three year old female child with a three month history of a limp. She was noted to be fretful and cried at nights. Clinically there was a flexion deformity of the right hip, muscle wasting in the right leg, restriction of movements in the right hip with pain at the extremes, and an increased lumbar lordosis.

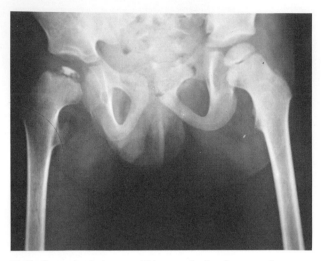

39. Radiograph ofasix year old boy wo had a three month
history of a painless limp. On clinical examination he was noted
to have marked restriction of internal rotation in the right hip.
There was no pyrexia, and the white blood count and
sedimentation rate were normal.

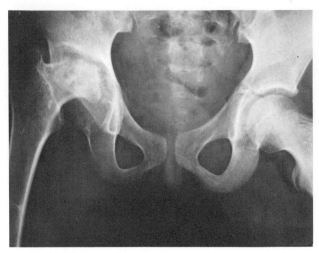

40. Radiograph of a 14 year old boy with a nine month history
of a limp, with progressive pain and stiffness in the right hip. He
was noted to have a fixed flexion deformity of the hip with an
associated increase in lumbar lordosis. Movements in the right
hip were grossly restricted, with pain at the extremes.

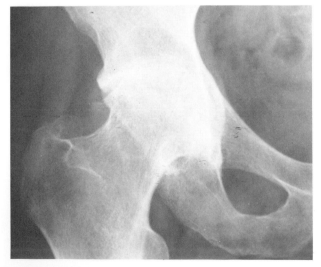

41. A-P radiograph of the hip of a 66 year old man who had
been complaining of increasing pain and stiffness in the joint over
the previous two years. He commented that he was unable to tie
his shoe laces or cut his toe-nails. There was no history of
previous trouble with the joint. He was noted to have marked
restriction of all movements in the hip (especially rotation), with
pain at the extremes.

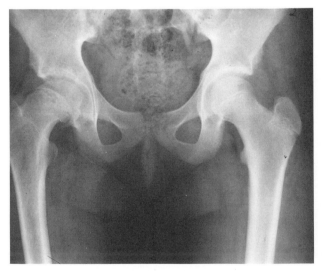

42. A-P radiograph of the hips of a plump 14 year old boy
complaining of mild pain and stiffness in the right hip, present
for two weeks. He walked with an obvious limp, and there was
restriction of rotation in the joint. The white blood count and
sedimentation rate were normal.

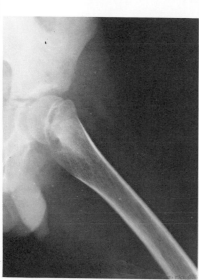
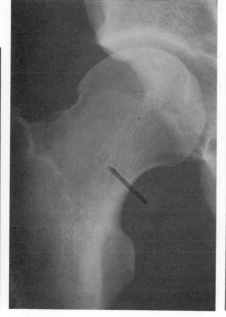
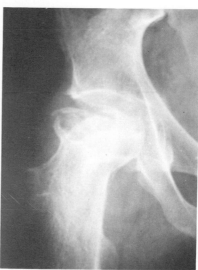

43. Lateral radiograph of 13 year old boy whose history and clinical findings were similar to the preceding case.

44. A 22 year old man complained of quite severe tooth-ache like pain in the right hip, present for ten months. Apart from some tenderness below the groin, no abnormality was found clinically; he had a full range of painless movements in the hip, and the ESR was normal.

45. Radiograph of a 30 year old man with a history of a fracture of the femoral neck two years previously. The nail used for fixation had been removed. He was complaining of pain in the hip, and gave a history of poliomyelitis in childhood.

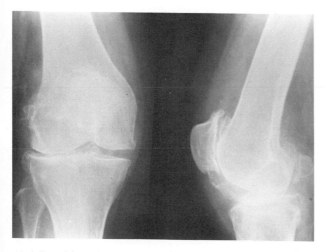
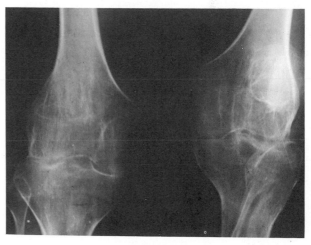

46. A-P and lateral radiographs of the right knee of a 68 year old retired labourer who was complaining of pain and stiffness in the joint. On examination he was found to have a slight fixed flexion deformity of the joint, a small effusion, limitation of flexion to 100°, and very marked crepitations on flexion and extension.

47. Radiographs of the knees of 30 year old man complaining of increasing pain and stiffness over the last two years. At the time of his attendance virtually no movements were detectable in the joints. He complained of general malaise, and his sedimentation rate was 95 mm in one hour. Further examination revealed marked restriction of movements in the spine.

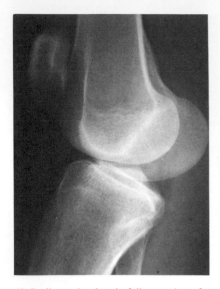

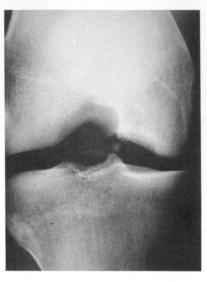

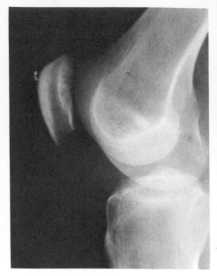

48. Radiograph taken in full extension of an 18 year old girl complaining of pain and clicking sensations in the right knee. Passive movements of the patella pressed against the femur gave rise to pain. Attempts to displace the patella laterally gave rise to apprehension.

49. Intercondylar view of the right knee of a 14 year old boy who had been complaining for some months of recurrent aching and swelling. A small effusion was present, and tenderness was observed over the medial femoral condyle.

50. A 23 year old woman gve a 2 year history of ill-localised pain at the front of the right knee, with frequent swelling of the joint. An effusion was confirmed clinically, and the articular surface of the patella was tender. Patellar movements were painful.

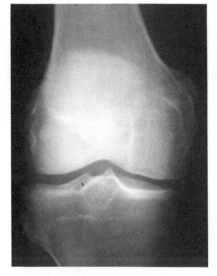

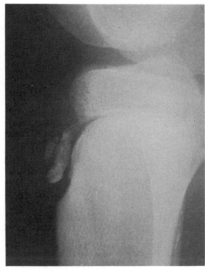

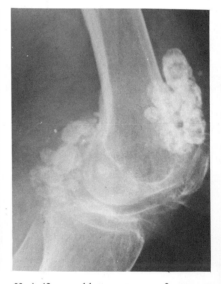

51. A-P radiograph of the knee of a 50 year old woman with a 6 month history of pain on the medial side of the joint. She was found to have well localised tenderness over the upper attachment of the medial ligament which however proved to be intact on testing.

52. Lateral radiograph of the knee of a 15 year old boy who was complaining of pain over the tibial tubercle, which on clinical examination was very prominent and tender. Symptoms had been present for 4 months, and there was no systemic disturbance.

53. A 42 year old woman gave a 2 year history of swelling, pain, giving way and occasional locking of the right knee. There was a gross effusion, quadriceps wasting, and synovial thickening. Small mobile masses were palpable in the suprapatellar pouch.

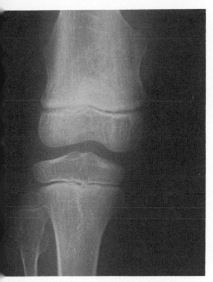

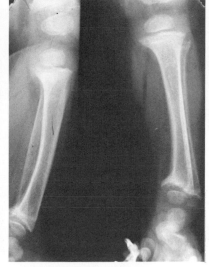

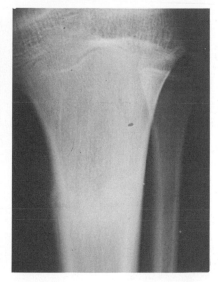

4. A 16 year old boy complained of a
~ainless swelling on the medial side of the
~g just below the knee—first noticed
~ome months before, but probably present
~uch longer. A similar swelling, arising
~om the tibia was found on the other side.

55. Radiographs of a 4 year old girl who
was noted to have lateral bowing of both
legs. The malleoli appeared unduly
prominent, and there was similar
thickening present above both wrists. The
serum calcium and phosphate were
respectively 2.14 and 1.1 u/mol/litre.

56. A 19 year old amateur rugby player
gave an 8 week history of left shin pain.
He was unable to recall any particularly
severe local trauma. On clinical
examination he was found to have well
localized tenderness and oedema over the
proximal tibia.

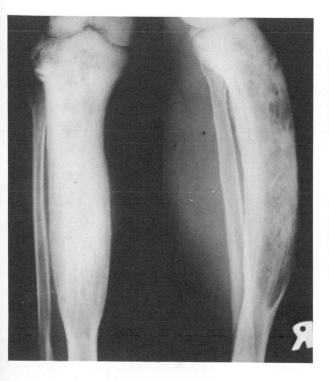

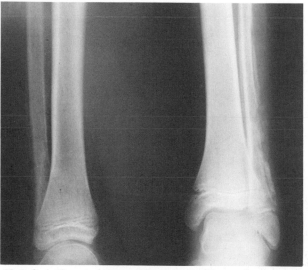

57. *Left:* A 58 year old man gave an 8 year history of
intermittent pain in the right shin which had a very marked
anterior curvature. The serum calcium and phosphate were
normal, but the alkaline phosphatase was raised. 58. *Above:* An
11 year old boy gave a 5 week history of pain and swelling of the
left leg, and inability to weight bear. At the onset there had been
high fever and positive blood culture.

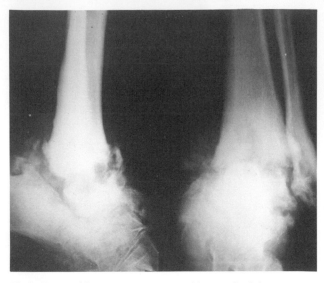

59. A 45 year old man gave a one year history of painless swelling and deformity of the left ankle. The ankle was found to be swollen and flail. The lower limb reflexes were absent and the pupils failed to respond to light. No sugar was detected in the urine.

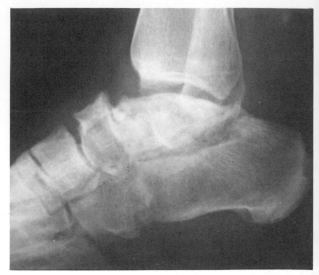

60. A 40 year old man complained of increasing pain in the right ankle following an injury which had been treated elsewhere. Details were incomplete, but he was believed to have sustained a dislocation of the talus. The foot and ankle were found to be swollen. Movements in both the ankle and sub-talar joints were greatly restricted and painful.

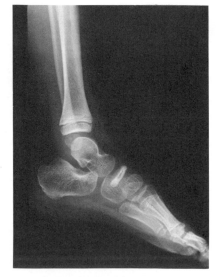

61. Lateral radiograph of a six year old boy who had been complaining for several months of aching pain on the medial side of the foot and an occasional limp. There was tenderness on the medial side of the foot, with pain on forced inversion.

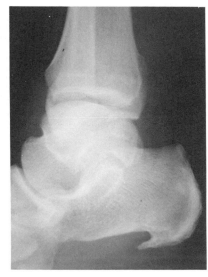

62. Lateral radiograph of a 57 year old man with a 4 month history of pain in one heel. There was marked local tenderness on the medial and inferior aspects of the heel.

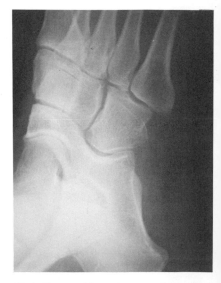

63. A 19 year old youth gave a 6 month history of pain in the right foot and a limp. The foot was held in eversion with flattening of the medial longitudinal arch. The ankle had a normal range of movements, but no inversion seemed possible.

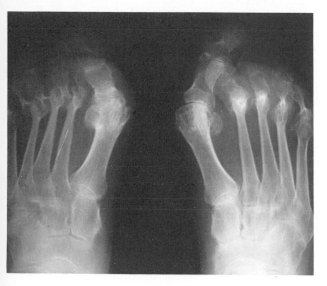

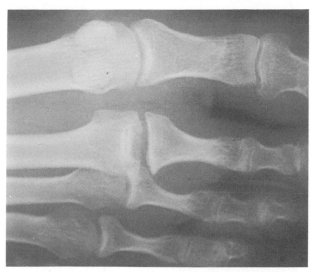

64. A 62 year old woman complained of pain under the metatarsal heads and of difficulty in obtaining comfortable shoes. She had multiple deformities including bilateral hallux valgus with over-riding second toes, splayed feet, and callosities under the metatarsal heads. The feet were warm to touch.

65. An 18 year old girl gave a three month history of pain in the right forefoot. She was noted to have some swelling on the dorsum of the foot at the base of the second toe. Tenderness was found at the same site. There was restriction of movements at the MP joint, and plantar-flexion was particularly painful.

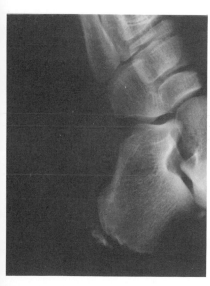

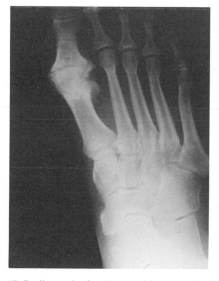

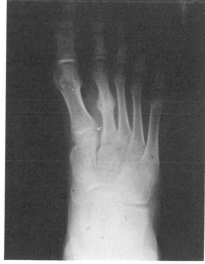

66. A 6 year old boy gave a six week history of pain in the left heel. He was found to have tenderness over the posterior aspect of the heel in the region of the insertion of the Achilles tendon.

67. Radiograph of a 45 year old man with a two year history of pain in the right great toe. There was no history of trauma or other joint involvement. The MP joint was palpably thickened and there was marked restriction of plantar and dorsi flexion.

68. A probationer nurse gave a four week history of fore-foot pain. She had no history of injury, but was found to have some pitting oedema and tenderness on the dorsum of the foot. Tenderness was also noted on palpation of the sole.

Answers and References

The cervical spine (p. 13)

1. Cervical spondylosis (Fig. 25). Note anterior lipping and narrowing of the C4-5 space.

2. Cervical spondylosis (Figs 25, 29). There is gross anterior lipping with some distortion of the pharyngeal shadow.

3. Atlanto-axial subluxation (Fig. 27) secondary to rheumatoid arthritis, with cord compression. There are widespread arthritic changes throughout the cervical spine.

4. Cervical tuberculosis (cervical caries) involving C1 and C2 (Figs 23, 29). Note the presence of a retro-pharyngeal abscess.

5. Subluxation of C3 on C4 (Figs 22, 24) with unilateral facet joint locking. Cervical spondylosis is also present.

6. Ankylosing spondylitis (Fig. 25). Note the widespread fusion of the facet joints, and calcification of the anterior longitudinal ligament.

The shoulder (p. 22)

7. Calcifying supraspinatus tendinitis (Fig. 39). Note the large mass of calcified material in the region of the greater tuberosity.

8. The radiograph shows the presence of an acromio-clavicular subluxation (Fig. 46).

The elbow (p. 34)

9. The radiograph shows an atrophic dislocated radial head and deformity of the ulnar shaft characteristic of an old unreduced Monteggia fracture (Fig. 31M). Tardy ulnar nerve palsy may follow both cubitus varus and valgus deformities.

10. Myositis ossificans (Fig. 32O).

11. Osteochondritis dissecans of the capitulum (Fig. 31J).

The wrist (p. 43)

12. Kienbock's disease of the lunate (Fig. 52H).

13. Metacarpal enchondroma (p. 58). The diagnosis was confirmed histologically after the swelling had been excised, curetted, and packed with bone chips.

14. Osteo-arthritis of the trapezo-metacarpal joint, with lateral subluxation of the thumb metacarpal (p. 58).

The wrist (p. 43)

15. Infective arthritis of the wrist due to tuberculosis (Fig. 52L).

16. Sudeck's atrophy (p. 43). Note widespread carpal decalcification with 'moth eaten' appearance.

The wrist (p. 43)

17. Old un-united fracture of the scaphoid (Fig. 52G) with early radio-carpal osteo-arthritis: note the narrowing between the radial styloid and the distal scaphoid fragment.

18. Osteitis of the terminal phalanx, with extensive bone destruction (p. 59).

19. All three appearances are normal (Fig. 53) and are incidental findings.

20. Infective lesion of the spine, subsequently proved tuberculous. Note the slight narrowing between L2 and L3 (numbering from the last rib). There is a faint abscess shadow in the upper part of the body of L3 (Fig. 55).

21. Senile kyphosis (Fig. 51). Note the narrowed disc spaces and anterior arthritic lipping.

22. Spina bifida occulta (Fig. 62) involving L5 and the sacrum

23. Congenital scoliosis due to hemivertebra (Fig. 63). There is an extra rib attached to the half segment.

24. Ankylosing spondylitis (Figs 66, 67). Note obliteration of sacro-iliac joints, interspinous ligament ossification and early bambooing. Pulmonary tuberculosis is not infrequently seen complicating ankylosing spondylitis.

The thoracic and lumbar spine (p. 71)

25. Vertebra plana (Calvé's disease) due to eosinophilic granuloma (Fig. 56). Note the preservation of disc spaces above and below the collapsed vertebral body.

26. Pathological anterior wedge compression fracture of D9 (Fig. 52) secondary to osteomalacia.

27. Scheuermann's disease of the spine (Fig. 51). Note the slight anterior wedging, irregularity of disc margins, and central disc prolapse.

28. Idiopathic scoliosis with primary curve from D5–D11 (Fig. 76).

29. Tuberculosis of the dorsal spine (Fig. 64). Note the loss of disc space, slight lateral wedging, and large paravertebral abscess.

30. Spondylolisthesis of L5 on S1. (Figs 70–74) with a little less than 25 per cent forward slip. The defect in the pars interarticularis is obvious in the lateral view, and in the oblique projection the corresponding 'Scotch terrier' or 'Scotty dog' has been decapitated.

31. Infective arthritis of the right sacro-iliac joint, subsequently proved to be staphylococcal in origin (Fig. 67).

The thoracic and lumbar spine (p. 71)

32. The radio-opaque medium is indented by a space occupying lesion on the right side, confirmed at surgery to be a prolapsed intervertebral disc (Fig. 81). The L5 nerve root was stretched over the disc mass on the right side.

33. Impacted fracture of the neck of the right femur (Fig. 64, E, F). Note the disturbance of Shenton's line.

The hip (p. 103)

34. Congenital dislocation of the left hip (Fig 87). Note the small capital epiphysis on the left side, its abnormal position in Perkins' square, and the high slope of the acetabulum.

35. Congenital coxa vara (Fig. 64G).

36. Congenital dislocation of the hip. On the left side the hip is dislocated, and the femoral head, femoral shaft and acetabulum are atrophic. On the right side the acetabular angle is increased, and the femoral head incompletely contained in the acetabulum (Dysplastic hip) (Figs 64D, 87).

37..Coxa valga (Fig. 64H).
   Atrophy of the right hemipelvis.
   Atrophy of the right femoral shaft.

38. Tuberculosis of the right hip. Note the acetabular irregularity and surrounding osteoporosis (Fig. 63, 64C).

39. Perthes' disease of the right hip. Note the increased density of the capital epiphysis (Fig. 63H) increased joint space (Fig. 69) and widening of the metaphysis (Fig. 71).

40. Infective arthritis of the hip with gross destruction (Fig. 64C) proved due to tuberculosis.

41. Osteo-arthritis of the hip (Fig. 67). Note the narrowed joint space with some marginal sclerosis. The line of the acetabulum is encroaching the inner wall of the pelvis. (Early protrusio-acetabuli — Fig. 66A).

42. Slipped femoral epiphysis (Figs 73, 74).

43. Slipped femoral epiphysis (Fig. 72).

The tibia (p. 156)

44. Osteoid osteoma (Fig. 16F). Note the small circular lesion with a central nidus in the femoral shaft on the same level as the lesser trochanter.

The hip (p. 103)

45. Segmental avascular necrosis of the femoral head (Fig. 63G). Note the marked superior segmental flattening and distortion. The fracture, just detectable by the kink in the medial part of the femoral neck, is soundly united as is usual. There is gross coxa valga (Fig. 64H).

The knee (p. 125)

46. Osteo-arthritis. Note (a) joint space narrowing (Fig. 98D) particularly of the patello-femoral and lateral compartments. (b) Arthritic lipping, especially of the patella, medial femoral condyle and lateral tibial table (Fig. 98E). (c) A small loose body visible in the A-P view in the medial compartment (Fig. 98H). (d) A large fabella is present (Fig. 97, 98A).

47. Ankylosing spondylitis (p. 73). Note obliteration of joint space and early bony ankylosis.

48. The radiograph shows a highly placed patella secondary to a moderate degree of genu recurvatum (Fig. 101). The findings suggested early recurrent dislocation of the patella and chondromalacia patellae.

The knee (p. 125)

49. Osteochondritis dissecans of the medial femoral condyle (Fig. 99) with separation of the fragment to form a loose body.

50. Chondromalacia patellae. Note the irregularity of the posterior aspect of the patella. A similar appearance was found in the tangential projection (Fig. 100).

51. Pellegrini-Stieda disease (Fig. 98J). Note calcification at the upper pole of the medial ligament.

The tibia (p. 156)

52. Osgood Schlatter's disease (Fig. 16B).

53. Synovial chondromatosis (p. 132). Note multiple loose bodies in the suprapatellar pouch and popliteal recess.

The tibia (p. 156)

54. Diaphyseal aclasis (Fig. 16A). Note involvement of both tibia and fibula.

The tibia (p. 156)
The knee (p. 125)

55. Rickets (Figs 14, 46A). Note the widening of the metaphyses at both ends of the tibia with characteristic cupping.

The tibia (p. 156)

56. Stress fracture of the tibia (Fig. 16C). Note increased bone density in the line of the fracture and the periosteal reaction on the medial side of the tibia.

57. Paget's disease. Note the characteristic alteration in bone texture (Fig. 15A). There was no evidence of sarcomatous change.

58. Osteitis of the fibula (Fig. 16D). Note the extensive destruction of bone and sub-periosteal new bone formation. A penicillin resistant staphylococcus aureus was grown on blood culture.

59. Charcot's disease. The Wassermann reaction was positive. Note the gross disorganisation typical of a neuropathic joint.

The ankle (p. 162)

60. Avascular necrosis of the talus. Note the bony collapse and secondary deformity (Fig. 37I).

61. Köhler's disease of the navicular (Fig. 108).

62. The radiograph shows a calcaneal spur (Fig. 112A) which is often found in association with plantar fasciitis (although not necessarily closely related to that condition).

63. Calcaneo-navicular synostosis (Fig. 115).

The foot (p. 173)

64. Rheumatoid arthritis (Fig. 107). Note multiple dislocation of the toes at the M.P. joints.

65. Freiberg's disease (Fig. 106B).

66. Sever's disease (Fig. 112). Note the increased density and fragmentation of the calcaneal epiphysis.

67. Hallux rigidus (Fig. 106C). Note the joint space narrowing and arthritic lipping.

68. March fracture (Fig. 106A).

Index

Numbers in italics refer to radiographs